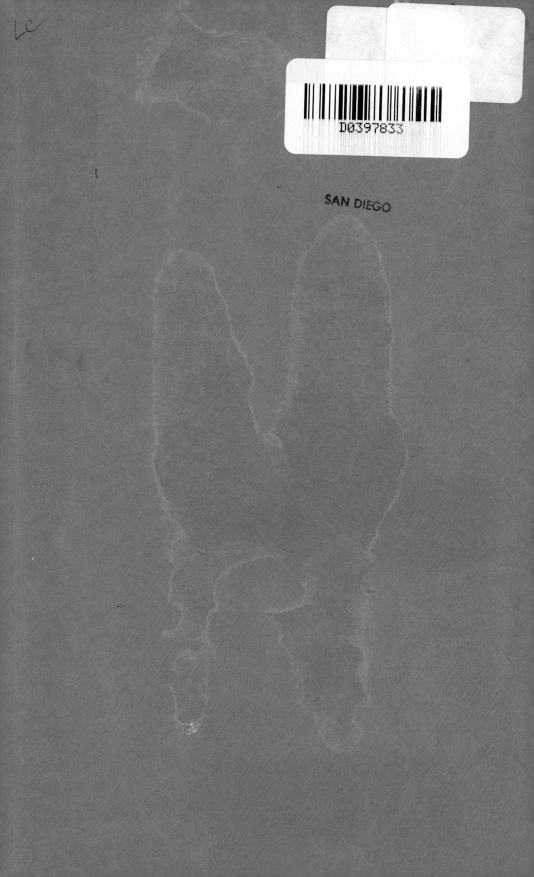

Forever
Young

ALSO BY STUART M. BERGER, M.D.

Divorce Without Victims
Southampton Diet
Dr. Berger's Immune Power Diet
Stuart Berger's Immune Power Cookbook
How to Be Your Own Nutritionist
What Your Doctor Didn't Learn in Medical School

Forever Young

20 Years Younger in 20 Weeks

DR. BERGER'S STEP-BY-STEP REJUVENATING PROGRAM

STUART M. BERGER, M.D.

WILLIAM MORROW AND COMPANY, INC.
New York

Library of Congress Cataloging-in-Publication Data

Berger, Stuart.
    Forever young : 20 years younger in 20 weeks: Dr. Berger's
step-by-step rejuvenating program / Stuart M. Berger.
        p.   cm.
    Includes index.
    ISBN 0-688-08208-4
    1. Longevity.   I. Title.
RA776.5.B437   1989   89-2953
613—dc19   CIP

Printed in the United States of America

First Edition

1   2   3   4   5   6   7   8   9   10

BOOK DESIGN BY BERNARD SCHLEIFER

For Marlaine, my best friend,
whose support is always
invaluable.

I want to express my gratitude to Pat Golbitz, Howard Kaminsky, Larry Hughes, Allen Marchioni, Lori Ames, and Carolyn Reidy, who represent the best in publishing.

To Lorna Darmour, Arthur Klebanoff, David Nimmons, and Marilyn O'Reilly for their knowledge, expertise, and dedication in completing this project.

A special thanks to Sally Jessy Raphael and Karl Soderlund for coming to me with this exciting idea.

And most of all to my parents, Otto and Rachel, who taught me the healing nature of laughter, and who are always there with love and support.

Contents

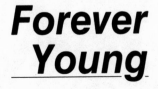

*Forever
Young*

1

Looking Forward to Getting Younger

THE SIXTEENTH CENTURY was a dozen years old or so when a Spanish galleon appeared off the coast of the Florida peninsula. On its decks, the famed Spanish explorer Juan Ponce de León sensed that he was within days of completing his sacred mission. As the ship rolled gently beneath his feet, he scanned the horizon. On those shores, he had heard tell, existed a secret fount. Revered by the Indians in the region, its waters had mysterious properties conferring lasting vigor, beauty, and youth to all who drank them. His quest, he knew, was to claim that fountain for Spain's king, Ferdinand II, and to bring that elixir home for the royal families of Europe.

Four centuries later, in a laboratory outside Miami, a white-coated cell biologist straightens up from her computer terminal. On its green phosphor screen, she has been mapping the very secrets that the Spanish explorer had dreamed of. Her quest focuses, not on the flowing waters of a mythical fountain, but on much more intimate ones: the biochemical fluids locked within the human immune cell. It is in these waters, she knows, that the real secrets of aging are to be found, etched in a complex code of DNA.

The book you hold in your hands is the culmination of a journey begun long ago, well before Ponce de León. It represents a dream that has tempted the human species ever since we lived in caves—the dream of a life without aging, without senescence or decay, where we stay forever young (well, *almost* forever—but then again, who wants to live to be 647 years old, anyway?).

Throughout human history, prolonging youth has been the province of magic and myth. Today, in the final decade of the twentieth century, it has become one of science and certainty. For the first time ever, we have the opportunity to realize that dream.

> Aging, as we have always known it, may no longer be in-evitable or irrevocable. Breakthroughs all across the fron-tier of biomedical science make it increasingly feasible to hope that we may hold back the ravages of senescence—even to abolish many of the degenerative symptoms of the hitherto-universal disease called old age. For nearly every symptom of aging . . . there are remedies and preventive measures being actively investigated.
> —ALBERT ROSENFELD, in *Prolongevity*

Today, thanks to research developments in the last decade, the deepest secrets of biological aging lie within our grasp. Again and again in these pages, you will find yourself confronting one central truth: *We now know enough to alter significantly the course of how—and how fast—we age.* Ours is the first generation that has a very real, very practical chance of staying younger, longer, than ever before. That is a chance you must be willing to take, or you would not have purchased this book.

A decade ago this book could not have been written, for many of the specific steps we will cover were then unknown. I can sit down to write it today because now we hold hard medical science in hand, promising and fascinating nuggets buried in papers from research labs the world over. Some of these steps may seem fa-miliar, others will be completely new to you. But by combining them all together in one cohesive program, you will realize all of the advantages that medical science can provide. You will have a simple, stepwise program to put these principles to work in your own life—starting this minute.

How realistic is that? Well, according to one eminent specialist on the aging process, writing in the *Proceedings of the National Academy of Sciences,*

> It is not unreasonable to expect on the basis of present data that the healthy life span can be increased by 5–10 or more years. . . .

That is our task in the pages that follow. You and I will bring those discoveries out of cloistered biochemistry laboratories and into your life—so you can begin to benefit from what scientists have pieced together. We will see what is surely the most exciting series of breakthroughs of the age, discoveries that go beyond simply unraveling any one disease or condition. Rather, these scientific advances address the whole spectrum of changes that occur—in our brains and biochemistry, in our cells and synapses—as our bodies age. Correctly and judiciously applied, the specific techniques in these pages are a prescription for remaining vital, healthy, and active until the very end of a long, productive life.

Welcome—to the Longevity Revolution

The prescription you are about to write for yourself draws from a diverse range of topics and disciplines: medicine, nutrition, immunology, cancer prevention, even exercise physiology. For what has happened in the last few years—and the main reason I could write this book—is that a number of scientific disciplines have converged. As that has happened, we have undergone what many call the "Longevity Revolution."

For many years, researchers in these fields had labored in relative isolation. Like so many blind men describing the same elephant, each beheld a small piece: aging as it happened in the cardiovascular system and the immune system, bone and skeletal changes, the chronological development of the brain.

But then, as laboratory scientists and clinical practitioners began to share information across disciplines, they started to find common ground, realizing that in many respects they were working on different pieces of the same vast puzzle. Their work started to coalesce; findings piled upon findings, reinforcing, substantiating, proving and disproving. Piece by painstaking piece, enough information has been assembled from medical science to make possible a book like this, dedicated to putting all of these findings in one place, with one common goal: keeping you younger.

Hardly a month goes by that I do not read of yet another research report, another vital piece of the puzzle about how we can slow—even, in some cases, reverse—the cellular processes of decay. The concrete signs of the pace of research in this area abound:

—The budget of the National Institute on Aging will reach an impressive $194 million this fiscal year, funding some 697 separate research projects.
—America now boasts some dozen scientific institutions devoted solely to anti-aging research and study.
—If you go to the nearest medical research library, you will find more than thirty-four journals devoted to findings on various aspects of aging—and aging prevention.

When I sat down to write this book, my first step was to key into a medical research computer bank the broad topic of "aging research." The answer it gave me testifies to the meteoric growth in this field—it selected more than 45,000 scientific papers for me to review!

All of this points in one very hopeful direction. We are now able to lengthen our lives, prolong our healthy and vital years, and reduce the procession of chronic, debilitating illnesses that have come to define old age. We have inched forward in our understanding of just what aging is, how it works, and—most important of all—what *you* can do about it.

"Youth Preservation": A Science Is Born

It is at this fertile crossroad that the science of "Youth Preservation" has come into being. Or at least, that's the term I use for it. Unfortunately, you will not yet find those exact words listed in the curricula at medical schools or in official proceedings. It remains a hybrid field, a mosaic of cell biology, genetics, biochemistry, oncology, geriatrics, and several other disciplines. But although we don't yet have an agreed-upon name for this science, it is clear that each of these disciplines is a part of the larger picture, and that this larger picture points the way to a younger, more vital you.

A certain part of this revolution is as simple as the fact that we have grown much more skilled at preventing a whole family of specific diseases of old age. It is a biological fact that just a handful of diseases—cancer, coronary artery disease, stroke, diabetes, kidney failure, obstructive lung disease, pneumonia, and the flu account for 85 percent of the debilitating illnesses of old age. Heart disease all by itself accounts for fully one out of every two deaths of older Americans, and high blood pressure directly causes or contributes to 15 percent of all deaths.

Yet amazingly, we can already control many of these diseases. Listen to the expert testimony of former Secretary of Health, Education and Welfare Joseph A. Califano, Jr., before the United States Senate:

"67% of all disease and premature death is preventable."

—Dr. Peter Greenwald, director of Cancer Prevention and Control at the National Cancer Institute, says that 80 percent of cancer cases are linked to how we live our lives—so can be controlled.
—Margaret Heckler, former Secretary of Health and Human Services, says, "Changes in lifestyle and behavior could save 95,000 lives per year by the year 2000."

What these experts are telling us is clear: If you did nothing else but focus on these high-risk diseases—by knowing how to eat, exercise, and live your life so you can lower your risk for them—you would automatically improve your odds for a reprieve from the most common, and obvious, causes of debility, premature aging, and death.

Research shows again and again that many of the problems we have come to expect as part of "just getting old" have more to do with *how* we live than how *long*.

—Coronary artery disease accounts for half of all deaths in those over sixty-five. But there is clear research showing that athero-

sclerosis—the artery clogging that is the main culprit in premature heart disease—is not a necessary part of aging. In most
mammals, and even in some human societies, it doesn't happen.
In Chapter 6 I give you six "young-at-heart" guidelines to make
sure it won't happen to you either.

—High blood pressure, as any doctor in this country will tell you,
rises with age—a rise of about 15 percent is considered "average."
But among the inhabitants of Easter Island, these changes in blood
pressure don't happen. Clearly, if they can avoid this damaging
rise, we can too.

—Bone weakening (osteoporosis) causes 1.2 million hip fractures every
year among older women, and some 40,000 deaths. Yet in China
and Japan, such fractures are extremely rare—because of factors
like diet and exercise. We will review the four crucial bone builder
tips in Chapter 8.

In these cases, as in many others, the more we look, the more
we see that many of the diseases we associate with age are highly
avoidable. As we add more diseases, one by one, to the list of
those we can most likely avoid, we tip the balance in our favor to
live longer, more active lives.

Family Health History Quiz

To understand what these specific discoveries may mean for
you, take a moment to do the following exercise. It is most appli-
cable if you are in your midthirties or above.

If you have lost parents, grandparents, or other older relatives, consider a few simple questions:

What did you father die from?   _____

What did your mother die from?   _____

What did your grandfather die from?   _____

What did your grandmother die from?   _____

What have other older relatives died from? _____

Without doubt, your list included such conditions as cancer,
heart disease, pneumonia, and infections. Now imagine how your

own medical future is changed by striking out those candidates from the list—because you have built them out of your life! By reducing your chances that those conditions will happen to you, you have already joined the Longevity Revolution!

Outwitting Mr. Gompertz

How old are you? Older than thirty-five? If so, Benjamin Gompertz has some disturbing news for you. Gompertz was a British scientist, population expert, and statistician who lived and wrote in the early years of the nineteenth century. In a famous formulation, which has come to be known as Gompertz' Constant, he estimated that the probability of dying increases exponentially every year after age thirty-five. Scientists have relied on the Gompertz Constant for years as they attempt to push back the limits of aging and death.

Just three years ago, Nobel Prize-winning biochemist Linus

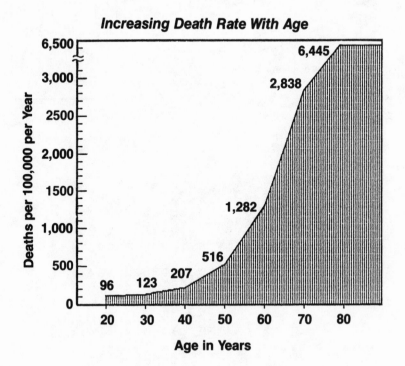

Increasing Death Rate With Age

Life Span According to State

Statistically, your chances for a long and healthy life vary significantly depending on where you live. Just for your information, you may find it interesting to find the average life span in your state:

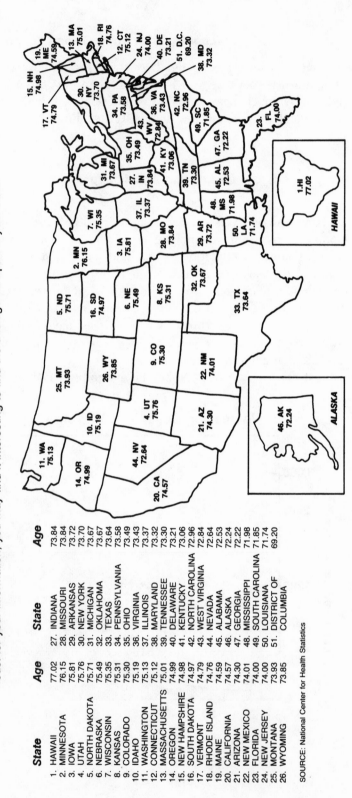

State	Age	State	Age
1. HAWAII	77.02	27. INDIANA	73.84
2. MINNESOTA	76.15	28. MISSOURI	73.84
3. IOWA	75.81	29. ARKANSAS	73.72
4. UTAH	75.76	30. NEW YORK	73.70
5. NORTH DAKOTA	75.71	31. MICHIGAN	73.67
6. NEBRASKA	75.49	32. OKLAHOMA	73.67
7. WISCONSIN	75.35	33. TEXAS	73.64
8. KANSAS	75.31	34. PENNSYLVANIA	73.58
9. COLORADO	75.30	35. OHIO	73.49
10. IDAHO	75.19	36. VIRGINIA	73.43
11. WASHINGTON	75.13	37. ILLINOIS	73.37
12. CONNECTICUT	75.12	38. MARYLAND	73.32
13. MASSACHUSETTS	75.01	39. TENNESSEE	73.30
14. OREGON	74.99	40. DELAWARE	73.21
15. NEW HAMPSHIRE	74.98	41. KENTUCKY	73.06
16. SOUTH DAKOTA	74.97	42. NORTH CAROLINA	72.96
17. VERMONT	74.79	43. WEST VIRGINIA	72.84
18. RHODE ISLAND	74.76	44. NEVADA	72.64
19. MAINE	74.59	45. ALABAMA	72.53
20. CALIFORNIA	74.57	46. ALASKA	72.24
21. ARIZONA	74.30	47. GEORGIA	72.22
22. NEW MEXICO	74.01	48. MISSISSIPPI	71.98
23. FLORIDA	74.00	49. SOUTH CAROLINA	71.85
24. NEW JERSEY	74.00	50. LOUISIANA	71.74
25. MONTANA	73.93	51. DISTRICT OF COLUMBIA	69.20
26. WYOMING	73.85		

SOURCE: National Center for Health Statistics

Pauling reexamined Gompertz's calculations and found that for most of us, the chance of death increases by almost 9 percent *each* year after age thirty-five.

Since your statistical chance of dying doubles every eight years and ten weeks, if you celebrated your thirty-fifth birthday today, that means the odds of your dying double by your forty-third birthday, and quadruple by your fifty-second birthday!

But there is a silver lining to this gloomy Gompertzian cloud. These numbers, remember, are based on an actuarial average. By the very act of picking up this book, and of launching yourself into a Youth Preservation Program, you are leapfrogging ahead of the population on whom such predictions are based. The many specific steps throughout this book help you take strong, positive action to outwit Mr. Gompertz's dismal numbers—and stay forever young.

The Longevity Revolution comes not a moment too soon. More people can benefit from such research than ever before—for the very simple reason that never before has our country had so many people getting older. Look around you. Statistics reflect that fact from every corner:

—This April, the U.S. Census Bureau reported that the nation's median age is at its highest point since they began tracking it 160

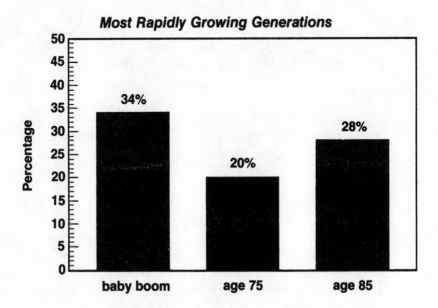

Most Rapidly Growing Generations

years ago. Today, one American in eight is over sixty-five—some thirty-two million people. That number is greater than the entire population of Australia, Belgium, and Israel combined! By the year 2030, the number will have doubled, to sixty-five million, or one American in five.

—The fastest-growing population segment is the baby boom generation, now aged thirty-five to forty-four. Next come seniors, seventy-five and older.

Still not convinced? Then just look at the shape of things to come, according to the National Institute on Aging:

Population Growth of Americans 85 years and Older

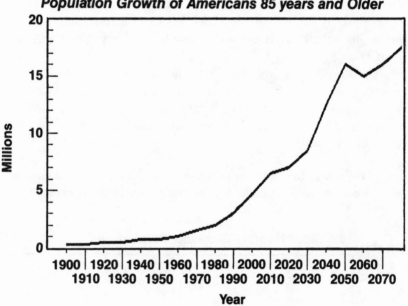

Such clear pictures are worth thousands of erudite words. The trend to an entire society living longer is unprecedented in our history—or, for that matter, in the history of the human race.

Not Just How Long, How Well

A major objective now and in the future should be maximizing health and well-being . . . so as to make life worth living for as long as possible. This will require a more careful application of preventive medicine."—DR. DENHAM HAR-MAN, biochemical gerontologist

"Adding life to years, not just years to life, is the goal of aging research."—DR. EDWARD SCHNEIDER, Dean, Gerontology Center, University of Southern California

Of course, there's more to longevity than just the sheer number of years you can manage to squeeze out. What counts as much—or more—is their quality. Those of us under sixty—the group in which you count yourself, I suspect—face a fundamental question: What quality of life can we look forward to? Do we intend to spend our later years in a twilight existence of failing health and vitality, paying the medical price for having ignored fundamental biological verities during our first half century, or will we take steps to transform ourselves into a culture of the healthiest, most youthful septuagenarians the world has ever known, able to take for granted the verve and vitality that is now associated with people ten, twenty, even thirty years younger?

I hear these questions being asked—and answered—every day. Many of my acquaintances, members of the baby boom, are just starting to feel the encroaching nibbles of age. Every day as I talk to patients and friends, as I lecture around the country and work with colleagues from New York to Hawaii, I become more convinced that the issue of what can be done to lengthen life and improve its quality is of unparalleled importance to the overwhelming majority of Americans.

What all of those people share—and this is true whether you are thirty-six or sixty-three—is a fervent desire to slow the rate at which their bodies are aging. Not just to live longer, but to live better. They seek a way to avoid the chronic diseases, encroaching fatigue, and degrading changes that seem to characterize old age. As a nation, we are looking to find what we can do to make our lives better, extend our most healthy, vibrant, active years, and shorten the time of weakness and failing health. We are a people ripe and ready to join the Longevity Revolution.

The goal is to put you on the dotted curve on page 26—to compress the time you spend ailing and frail, and extend the time you spend in full, robust, and energetic health.

For each of us, the realization of aging surfaces in different ways. Are you:

Two Views of Aging

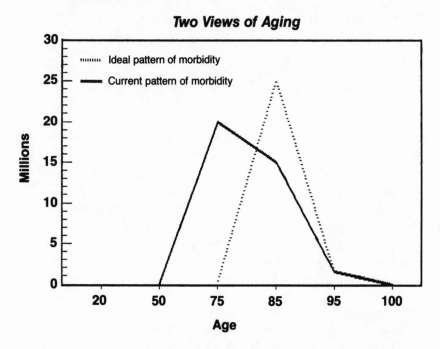

—Between twenty-five and thirty-five, just beginning to feel the first subtle twinges of growing older? You notice you sleep later on weekends than you once did. Maybe you can't stay out as late without feeling some ill effects. You may have watched your weight rise slightly, pounds getting easier to put on and harder to lose, as your metabolism changed. Perhaps sometime in the last year you suffered a minor sprain or injury in some athletic pursuit—an injury that you would have shrugged off five years ago.

—Between thirty-five and forty-five, having seen a friend, parent, or family member struck down with some serious disease? That experience may have made you start reading the health pages with a little extra care. Perhaps your doctor has found a condition like heart disease, diabetes, or obesity that "bears watching." Or maybe you are a parent, enjoying the new life you have brought into the world, but being reminded that you have a finite amount of time left in your own life.

—Between fifty-five and sixty-five? You may feel in good shape, but have started to take a certain amount of impairment for granted? You tire more easily, and have grown used to living with the arthritis, or gout, or heart condition your doctor diagnosed. You cannot help but hope that you will avoid the seriously deteriorating health that seems to have overtaken many of your contemporaries. You want to make sure you spend your next years enjoying what you have worked for instead of fighting discomfort, decay, and disease.

If you see yourself described here, or if you have simply wondered if there isn't something you ought to be doing to increase your health and longevity, I think you will find much to interest you in the pages that follow.

Among the important breakthroughs you will discover in these chapters:

—Your own health and life-style test to help you design an anti-aging program that is just right for you (Chapter 4)

—How you can best use the newest anti-aging skin-care treatments (Chapter 5)

—The nutritional keys you can use *now* to decrease the aging of your skin (Chapter 5)

—The just-discovered nutrient that promises a bone-rejuvenation breakthrough (Chapter 8)

—A specific nutritional plan to take you off the danger list for cardiac problems (Chapter 6)

—The effect that one simple change may have on reversing skeletal aging (Chapter 8)

—The "Antiviral Cocktail," first developed for AIDS, that can help increase your immune strength (Chapter 9)

—The safe vitamin treatment your doctor can give you to help restore your immune system to its youthful vigor (Chapter 9)

—The simple principles you can use to keep your brain younger, longer (Chapter 10)

—The dietary key to reducing the cellular changes leading to old age, and an eating plan to help you use it (Chapter 11)

—The new findings about the difference between exercise and activity—and how they affect your longevity (Chapter 11)

—The one single change some of you can make that is *100 percent guaranteed* to extend your healthy lives (Chapter 7)

—A step-by-step plan to reprogram the internal computer that may be aging you prematurely (Chapter 13)

My 20-20 Pledge to You

In health there are no absolute guarantees. But by following the twenty-plus specific health counsels in these pages, I can assure you that:

1. You will be following the best, most scientifically sound attempt you can make at present to stay younger, longer.
2. You will find them practical, real, do-able with inexpensive tools you have at your disposal.
3. By following these steps for twenty weeks, you will already feel and see a significant change in your appearance, health, and vitality.
4. The steps in these chapters will definitely help you feel better, with more energy and less likelihood of chronic disease.
5. By *not* heeding these principles, you will certainly shorten your healthy, productive life span.

I hope you take the 20-20 pledge: *That by following the twenty-plus guidelines throughout this book, you feel better in twenty weeks—and could add up to twenty years of productive, healthy, vigorous life.*

In return, I have to ask for one promise: that you will do your best to start thinking differently. Like Ponce de León, you need to become something of an explorer. But unlike his fantastic quest, yours has a sure chance of success, for it is based on science, not on speculation.

Being an explorer means you will have to get used to a whole new way of thinking. Perhaps the most significant changes of aging happen, not in your arteries, muscles, and bones, but in that marvelous organ nestled between your ears. When it comes to Youth Preservation, it is clear that the biggest differences lie in the choices we make many times each day: decisions about what we will eat, how we move, how we treat ourselves, even what inner tapes we play as we drift to sleep at night. Being around enjoying life in thirty, forty, or fifty years means having a strong inner commitment to longevity, starting right now.

You may find that hard at first because we are all so conditioned to see our lives in terms of the allotted threescore years and ten. Society has accustomed us to expect to live that length of time and no more, and I believe that at a very profound level we actually "program" ourselves to make it come true. I'll get to the specifics in Chapter 13, but the main point to keep in mind as you read this book is that you may be called upon to make a radical shift in that "programming," in how you see your life now, where you are headed, and what your future will look like.

If you've thought of retirement, of dropping out and taking it easy, of "coasting out" your last golden decade and a half, you may find yourself wanting to reconsider. I hope you will come to see retirement as just one of your options, along with other scenarios that have you working productively and energetically, physically and mentally active for more years than you had ever dared hope.

That's the kind of thinking I hope you'll do a lot of throughout this book. Because if you conscientiously apply the principles in it, you'd better have a good plan for how you want to spend all that extra time you'll be building into your life!

More on this subject later, but for now I just ask you to keep your heart and mind open to changing the way you see yourself and your life path, and to consider that a work in progress as you read the pages ahead.

So if I have that promise from you, and you have these pledges from me, let us not waste another minute that you could be using to grow younger. Come along, and together we'll take up where Ponce de León left off and finish that noble quest begun so many centuries ago. I hope you *are* looking forward—to growing younger!

2

Fables, Fountains, and Facts

All the days of Methuselah were nine hundred sixty and nine years: and he died.
—GENESIS 5:27

Do not try to live forever; you will not succeed.
—GEORGE BERNARD SHAW

GEORGE BERNARD SHAW was right. Obviously, I can't promise you that after you read this book, you can look forward to an added nine centuries of life. (Even back in Methuselah's time, when miracles like burning bushes and parting seas were everyday occurrences, living to his ripe age of 969 was considered pretty out of the ordinary.) More common, according to the very next chapter of Genesis, was that Man's "days shall be an hundred and twenty years"—the very age, by coincidence, that Moses died.

It turns out that those biblical "biologists" were pretty accurate—even today, the biological maximum life of *Homo sapiens* is generally agreed by most aging experts to be in the range of 115 to 120 years. That may seem strange, at first. After all, how many people do you know who live to be 115? Well, the factor to keep in mind is that such a figure represents, not the average, but the likely utmost top limit. That number has not changed appreciably since ancient Rome, when Pliny the Elder wrote that centenarians were, if not common, not unknown either. He even described a popular actress who was then one hundred years old. Today, the oldest documented living person is 114 years old; the oldest person ever authenticated lived to the age of 120. And while biomedical science may succeed in pushing back that limit, extending the hypothetical upper limit is not the main focus of this book.

I hold a much more practical—and, I believe, more easily achieved—goal. Obviously, most of us don't live anywhere near our 115-year limit. What the biblical scholars estimated as three-score and ten has been refined by latter-day biostatisticians as 74.7 years—the average life expectancy today in America. But the real question is: What happens in that gap between 74.7 years and 115?

Closing the gap is what this book is all about. Together, we can give you the edge so that you can more fully achieve your inbred biological maximum. It is the same goal that Wilder Penfield, the famed American neurosurgeon, envisioned when he wrote that he foresaw a day when "more men and women reach life's true goal, fulfilling the cycle set for us, bypassing the plagues, disease and famine."

We want to take his advice, to *take maximum biological advantage* of the preset limit built into our body's aging time clock—and to do it in such a way that what time we do have will be the healthiest, happiest possible. We first need to know what aging really is—and that, in turn, means debunking a few fables about what it most certainly is not.

First, the Fables . . .

Through the centuries, mankind's preoccupation with the subject of aging has been matched only by its collective imagination in devising ways to deal with it. The history of Youth Preservation spans several millennia of wild expectations, dashed hopes, and failed promises.

Five thousand years ago, in the oldest tale of Western civilization, the Babylonians told of the king Gilgamesh, who wanted to live forever. To do so, he was told by a sage, he must eat a certain plant growing under water, whose powers "restore lost youth to a man. . . . By its virtue a man may win back all his former strength. Its name shall be 'The-Old-Men-Are-Young-Again.' " Gilgamesh vowed to eat it and "return to what I was in my youth."

While that may have been the first time this idea arose, it was certainly not the last. For thousands of years, across many of the world's great cultures, the quest continued. The Chinese, the ancient Hebrews, Greeks, and Romans, medieval monks and twentieth-century Swiss doctors, each offered their own unique contributions to the pursuit of elusive immortality. Several thousand years ago, Chinese apothecaries whipped up an anti-aging cocktail called "tan," compounded from gold and the mercury-containing ore cinnabar (given the proven toxic effects of both metals, it is likely this "youth-preserving" formula hastened the deaths of those who swallowed it).

The Taoist religion held as a central goal the prolonging of life through nutrition, meditation, sports, and even sex. In biblical times many Middle Eastern societies believed that living to a ripe old age was God's reward for right-living and faith. For them, the key to remaining youthful—or at least alive—was not an elixir, but one's behavior. Those fortunate few who lived long enough to show the effects of age—no scant feat in an era when most people died by age forty—were considered models of appropriate living, deserving honor and reverence by virtue of their longevity. The Arabs spoke of a Well of Life that, like Ponce de León's fountain two millennia later, would confer glorious youth on those who enjoyed its waters.

In Europe during the Middle Ages, the practice of alchemy held as a goal, not to turn lead into gold—as is popularly believed—but to create nostrums that would forestall aging. The topic continued to fascinate Europeans for several hundred years. One scholarly work, written in the sixteenth century, explained that aging was the result of the loss of "vital particles" that we exhale with each breath. The way to stay young, it suggested, had been discovered by the occupant of an ancient Egyptian tomb who had lived an impressive 115 years. According to the inscription on the burial vault, he owed his longevity to "the Breath of Young Women." A colorful prescription, to be sure (and one that more than a few of my male patients would gladly accept!), but hardly accurate.

In our own century, the quest has taken a more scientific turn. In the 1920s, it was believed that the secret to prolonging vigor in men at least was to transplant into them the testicles of virile apes. Needless to say, this fanciful treatment did not yield any positive results (but I can't help wondering if the elderly male patients showed any increased craving for bananas!).

During the next decade, longevity again captured the popular imagination, in the form of the immensely popular book *Lost Horizon*. The tale told of Shangri-La, a city high up in the mountains, where the secret to infinite youth was to be found.

Not long thereafter, this time in the mountains of Central Europe, a researcher named Ana Aslan discovered what she thought was the cure to aging. In the early 1950s, this Rumanian biochemist created a drug called Gerovital-H3, which she claimed would reduce the changes of aging. It set off a flurry of research, and scores of eager patients flocked from the world over to her clinic at the Geriatric Institute in Bucharest. Today, some thirty-five years later, research has shown that the initial hopes for the drug were overoptimistic, and that the drug does not have any significant antiaging effects.

Not far away, in Switzerland, you can still check into one of the most renowned (and expensive) clinics and be injected in the rump with a puree made from the cells of lamb fetuses. These cells are claimed to inspire your old decrepit cells to be younger—a dramatic notion, to be sure, but there is no evidence in any credible scientific journal to suggest it works.

In recent years the anti-aging doctors have trotted out an alphabet soup of different chemical compounds—BHT, SOD, L-DOPA, NDGA, to name a few—to chemically forestall the cellular damage of aging and so keep us younger. While several of these compounds initially appeared to show promise, none has given us the magic key to aging that their inventors hoped.

And Now, the Facts

After many long centuries of fanciful theorizing, it is only in the last few years that we have advanced to the point of pinning down the true causes and mechanisms of aging—and with them, the clues to staying young.

The rest of this chapter is dedicated to bringing you up to date on some of the most current thinking. I hope you'll read it because it will help you understand the rationale for the steps we will undertake together in later chapters—the self-help core of this book.

However, I understand that you may be a doer, not a student, and may be impatient to get started on your twenty-week plan for improving your health and extending your life. You may be less interested in the theory than in beginning your own specific anti-aging steps *now*. If that is you, you are welcome to skip the rest of this chapter and go directly to the next chapter, which begins the interactive self-assessment for your own Youth Preservation Program. But if you do that, promise me one more thing— you will come back and read this chapter later . . . please?

A key event happened in 1964 when a premier microbiologist named Leonard Hayflick made a basic but crucial discovery. The human cells he was looking at would divide only about fifty times, then die—and little could be done to change that pattern. Hayflick's discovery took us a major step forward because it focused the debate on aging away from the larger organ systems to the innermost workings of the body's trillions of cells. It became a cornerstone in the whole new scientific discipline of biogerontology, the biological study of aging.

Today it is a scientific truism that we will not understand aging until we understand the astoundingly complex mechanics that happen within our cells. However, if everybody agrees that the cell is the "scene of the crime," there is less accord about exactly what happens inside it when we grow older.

There is no shortage of theories. Look at a recent list compiled by the National Institute on Aging:

Wear-and-tear theory
Rate-of-living theory
Metabolic theory
Endocrine theory
Free-radical theory
Collagen theory
Somatic mutation theory
Programmed senescence theory
Error catastrophe theory
Cross-linking theory
Immunological theory
Redundant message theory

Codon restriction theory
Transcriptional event theory

Behind each of these intriguing names are learned scientists, thoughtful adherents, and detractors. To give you an idea of all those theories would require several volumes and a graduate course, and that is hardly our goal here. But it is useful to get a basic familiarity with a few of the most common theories, because it is on this work that much of this book is based.

Most of the backers of the prime theories fall into one of two broad camps: those I call the "Entropists" and those I term the "Genetic Fatalists."

The Entropy of Age

Newton's Second Law of Thermodynamics, known to physicists as "entropy," states that things cool off over time. Scientists tell us that means that any organized system tends to move from order to chaos. (Anyone who has ever seen my workdesk at home— or, for that matter, any parent who has tried to keep a child-filled household tidy—knows exactly what I'm talking about!)

The same principle of entropy holds true, too, at a biological level. Every living organism is engaged in a constant struggle with the forces of entropy and disorder. That struggle is what aging is. Not only do our cells, and organs, and functioning become more disorderly with every passing year, the fact is, we literally "cool off"—our body temperature will have dropped by an average of two degrees by age seventy! In a very real sense, being alive means being engaged in a constant struggle against disorder, and our final capitulation to chaos comes only when we expire.

There is a whole school of thought that relies on entropy as the most likely explanation of aging. The Entropists say that it is wear and tear, the accumulating clutter of living that does us in. They postulate that the aging of the body's cells is much like the decay of, say, an old barn. Little by little, different things break down, damaged by the ravages of time. A hinge may fail there, a coat of paint peel here, a window sag somewhere else, and *voilà*— soon we are experiencing the creaky, slow, throbbing decrepitude of old age.

Although experts agree that such a gradual process occurs, they do not all agree about where to place most of the blame. Some say the "scene of the crime" is DNA, the genetic code that lies at the heart of human cells. Because of exposure to toxins, chemicals and ultraviolet light filtering through the skin, these complex chains of information-carrying chemicals may break, twist, become transposed, or otherwise get out of order. When they do, goes the theory, the cells are not able to pass along their genetic blueprints accurately, and key chemical reactions within the body's cells begin to go haywire. When enough of these cells break down, the scientists hypothesize, the changes accumulate into serious deficits that weaken whole organs. It is an intriguing proof for this theory that those animals whose cells repair DNA damage quickly and efficiently are also those who live the longest.

Another theory focuses more on the enzymes our cells produce. Sometimes they become faulty, and instead of the well-ordered cellular chemical production lines that Nature designed, our cells start to look like a crazed, disorderly factory floor, turning out too much of some things and not enough of others.

Another popular theory that researchers have focused on has been termed the "error catastrophe" theory. It suggests that defective proteins in the body's cells accumulate into an intracellular chemical soup that interferes with the cells' proper biochemical tasks and thus weakens them. Others suggest it is not that the chemicals are made wrong, but that they never get broken down and recycled properly. The image these biologists paint is one in which the cells' "work space" grows increasingly chaotic because its "janitors" are out on strike.

A "Radical" Theory of Aging

The most compelling of the many aging theories advanced by cell biologists is called the "free-radical" theory. It is this theory that underlies many of the nutritional counsels throughout this book—and it plays a role in many of the twenty-four rejuvenation steps we will explore.

This dramatic-sounding name, with its overtones of terrorists and saboteurs, may remind you of something from political theory instead of biology. Indeed, from your cells' point of view, that is almost exactly right. *Free radicals* are very reactive chemical by-products that are created as oxygen is burned as fuel in our cells. (For that reason, chemists also know them as "oxidation products.") Chemically, they are molecules out of electrical balance. Unfortunately, the only way they know to rebalance themselves is to steal an electron belonging to another molecule, thereby unbalancing it. And so the chain reaction goes, unleashing all sorts of havoc.

Free radicals can interact with fatty molecules, lipids, in your cells. Then, they create a pollutant, a sort of intracellular sludge called "lipofuscin," a pigment that can change the color of skin. However, their damage is far more than cosmetic. As they react explosively with many of your cells' natural chemicals, these free-radical reactions can inflict severe damage on the fragile equilibrium of the cells. (In fact, the damage they do is the same that occurs when you are exposed to radiation—except it is happening all the time, from the inside, instead of from an external radiation source.)

Free radicals destroy key cell enzymes, fats, and proteins. If they borrow electrons from fat molecules in the critical membrane wall of a cell, they can actually destroy the integrity of the cell. Too, they can interfere with the elegant intermeshing ballet of DNA and RNA that is responsible for cell division. As these miscreants do their dirty work, trouble begins to spread far and wide. They can trigger inflammation, damage lung cells and blood vessels, and lead to mutations, cell destruction, degenerative diseases, and even cancer. In terms of the destruction they cause, free radicals are the biological equivalent of a terrorist bomber gone berserk in the control room of a nuclear reactor. As enough of the cells' vital mechanisms are damaged, the cell can become less efficient, malfunction, or even die.

And when enough of *that* happens, there is a cascade of biological damage. The cumulative levels of oxidation radicals put millions, even billions, of cells out of commission. As you read this sentence, free radicals are slowly building up and being destroyed in your body. But as you age, their numbers certainly increase, and as they do, the chances also increase that these cellular saboteurs can do greater and greater harm to the "works" of your cells.

One school of thought, based on the breakthrough research of the eminent biologist Dr. Denham Harman, believes that the cumulative effect of free-radical damage is the root of cell aging—and all the debilitating, difficult diseases that often come with increasing years. The researchers are quite unequivocal: "Chances are 99% that free radicals are the basis for aging," says biochemist Harman, the father of free-radical theory. "Aging is the ever-increasing accumulation of changes caused or contributed to by free radicals." These scientists blame free radicals for many common degenerative diseases: arthritis, diabetes, hardening of the arteries, heart and kidney ailments, Parkinson's disease, even cataracts. As I was writing this chapter, the largest group of free-radical scientists in history met in an international colloquium to review the newest findings about these agents—and how to disable them. You will find some of their findings—particularly those about antioxidant nutritional defenses—in the chapters to come.

HOW NOT TO BE NATURE'S GUINEA PIG

Why on earth would Mother Nature have evolved us to have such potentially damaging chemical reactions? Denham Harman suggests two reasons: First, the same free radicals that cause aging and cancer also make it possible for all of the biological mutations that Nature has used over billions of years to make you the terrific, nearly perfect person you are. You can thank free radicals for the fact that you no longer swing from trees and walk on all fours! In that respect, free radicals are biological wild cards, thrown in to keep the evolutionary game interesting and moving along.

Second, the fact that free-radical oxidation plays a part in aging and cancer "may play a useful role, possibly a necessary one . . . by aiding in the disposal of old organisms after they have provided new 'experiments' for evaluation against the environment." Gulp. We are, of course, the "old organisms" Harman is talking about. But just in case you don't like the idea of being one of Nature's guinea pigs as your free radicals run wild, you will find suggestions for a potent antioxidant plan in the twenty-two steps throughout this book.

Although scientists may disagree whether the aging culprit is DNA, free radicals, defective cell enzymes, or some combination of these and other factors, what links all of them is a belief that losing our youthful vigor is a process of entropy, the result of the wear and tear of existence. They tell us it is when our cells grow increasingly snarled, jumbled, and generally muddled with chemical clutter that we start to look, act, and feel old.

Old age is like a plane flying through a storm. Once you are aboard, there is nothing you can do.

—GOLDA MEIR

The second major school of theorists says there is more to aging than mere entropy. These scientists are the Genetic Fatalists, whose credo, as voiced by one of their proponents, runs: "Life is a terminal disease." Their idea is simple. The human body is programmed to self-destruct, and the code to do so is written in our genes.

A concise view of this theory was written by the eminent immunobiologist Lewis Thomas in his *Medusa and the Snail:* "This is . . . what happens when a healthy old creature, old man or old mayfly, dies. The dying is built into the system so that it can occur at once, at the end of a genetically pre-determined allotment of living."

The possibility of genetic programming certainly goes a long way to explaining why the human species seems to have a fixed upper age of about 115 years. That presumably represents the maximum age our genes are "set" to. The adherents of such a theory cite the evidence of evolution: In order to continue the species, humans need survive only about thirty years—just enough time to have children. From an evolutionary perspective, the following seventy years are just so much window dressing, which confers little survival advantage for the species. They cite, too, the fact that the way our bodies change as we age—even down to such physical changes as our ears lengthening and our noses widening—as evidence for cellular programming to distribute fat, connective tissue, and even bone mass differently. Why then, they ask, could we not also be programmed to expire?

Some experts postulate that certain organs or organ systems control the body's internal clock. Noting that the immune system loses 90 percent of its power between the ages of fourteen and seventy, many biogerontologists have suggested that this complex system of cells, organs, and chemical messengers may be the body's "longevity timer." Others point to one part of the immune system, the thymus gland, as our biological pacemaker. Whether the cause is to be found in the whole or the part, what seems clear is that when our immune system weakens past a certain point, we succumb to the cancer or infections which a younger person would fight off.

The pathologist Roy Walford, a preeminent researcher at the University of California at Los Angeles, believes that immune system decline is probably controlled by a group of genes with the tongue-twisting name of major histocompatibility complex—MHC, for short. The MHC may affect breakage and repair of DNA, the levels of free radicals, even the pace at which our tissues develop and regenerate.

I have even heard other researchers point out that what may seem like built-in immune programming to grow older may in fact be due to the foods we eat throughout our lifetime. They believe that our immune system can be overtaxed by creating antibodies to deal with the many foreign proteins in the foods we consume. In the long haul, they argue, a steady barrage of foreign substances exhausts our B cells, T cells, and the natural killer cells of our immune defenses so that eventually they become depleted and cannot rise to the challenge when we need them—to fight off infections and cancers.

Tower of Biological Babel?

By now, you may feel that you are listening to the tower of scientific babel—or do I mean babble?—and can't distinguish a word that seems helpful. When the truth is finally sorted out, it may turn out that both sides are right. Our species' upper age limit of 115 years may be set by genetic limits locked into our genes, but we may rarely reach it because of the daily wear and tear that damages our cells long before then.

For you, who just want to live better and longer, this is something of an abstract discussion. When the experts seem so far apart, postulating such disparate mechanisms as genetic programming, DNA damage, accumulated cell toxins, even the food we eat, how can you make sense of it all? After all, if we don't know just what causes aging, how can we slow the process down?

Although I would be the first to admit that we do not yet have the final theoretical answer, I hope you aren't feeling dismayed. There is a relatively easy answer here: What you need to keep in mind is that there are several quite clear things that are helpful to focus on.

If you can increase your life expectancy from the seventy-four years that the statisticians tell us is now the norm even *halfway* up to the theoretical current maximum of 115 years, you would lengthen your life by 27 percent—more than one quarter. This may sound like an ambitious goal—indeed it is. But it doesn't mean it is not practical. Linus Pauling, three-time Nobel Prize-winning biochemist, estimates in *How to Live Longer and Feel Better* that using health measures presently available, we can increase our life expectancy from twenty-five to thirty-five years. Gerontologists Denham Harman and Roy Walford have estimated the potential additional time as five to ten years, which gives us a life span of about eighty-five years. Even the august National Institute on Aging, a mainline institution if there ever was one, published a paper saying that certain interventions "can improve heart and lung function, staving off normal age-related decrements by as much as 10 years."

People in developed countries have already added an astounding twenty-eight years to their average life span since the beginning of the twentieth century. *There is no reason whatsoever for not continuing that progress,* extending your life span even further.

The major point to keep in mind is that such an increase requires no fundamental change in scientific understanding, no major conceptual breakthroughs of the sort that researchers work and worry over. It doesn't necessarily matter, in fact, *which* of the many theories ultimately prove right.

All that it requires is following the steps detailed throughout these chapters. As you do so, you will build risk factors and unnecessary toxins out of your life; you will give your cells a chance to rebuild themselves. Your goal is to eliminate the factors that could prematurely truncate your life long before its true biological deadline. By doing so, you will let your body take advantage of the wonderful longevity that Nature originally designed into it.

74—THE MAGIC NUMBER?

If you live to the age of a hundred, you have it made, because very few people die past the age of a hundred.

—GEORGE BURNS

There is a grain of truth to the venerable comedian's counsel. If you are about to celebrate your seventy-fourth birthday, don't dust off your will just yet. Yes, seventy-four may be the average age, but that is a statistical confusion. It really reflects the large numbers of people who die prematurely from diseases and accidents. The thing to keep in mind is that, if you are healthy enough to live to a healthy, vital seventy, the chances are you will live another decade longer!

The System Is the Secret

What has become increasingly clear is that the answer to staying young will be found, not in one magic bullet, but in a connected web of behavior—how we eat, sleep, work, exercise, even think. That understanding is the basis of the more than twenty longevity steps you will find throughout this book, and that together make up a "systems approach" to keep you young.

It was the famed British physician Sir James Crichton-Browne who wrote: "There is no short-cut to longevity. To win it is the work of a lifetime, and the promotion of it a branch of preventive medicine." I couldn't agree more, and it is that principle that underlies the changes I will be asking you to make in your life over the next twenty weeks.

I hope you don't see those twenty weeks as a shortcut to longevity—they are not. Instead, you should think of them as a training period, a time for you to explore, acquire, and learn the new habits that you will incorporate into your life and carry for a lifetime. If you do that, you will reap a handsome dividend in terms of the length, the quality, and the pure enjoyment of your years ahead.

3
The Changes of Aging

To me, old age is always fifteen years older than I am.
—Bernard Baruch

EVERY ONE OF your body's systems, from your hair to your toenails, will undergo predictable changes as you age.

To stay young and vital for as long as possible, you need some idea of what really happens as a body grows older (keep in mind this isn't just *any*body we're talking about—it's *your* body!). So put on your physician's white coat and let's look at the physiological changes that lie ahead for you. Only by understanding what Nature has in store for us can we hope to control the aging process.

"An adult is a person who has ceased to grow vertically, but not horizontally."

This change is called the "Great Metabolism Shift," and it starts somewhere around the beginning of your fourth decade. Your energy furnaces start to burn differently, and Nature begins to swaddle you with an extra layer of fat. As fat increases, you also lose lean muscle mass; so your fat-to-muscle ratio increases significantly over the years, as shown on the charts on page 46.

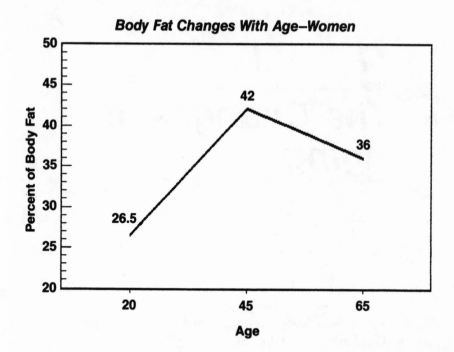

Body Fat Changes With Age–Women

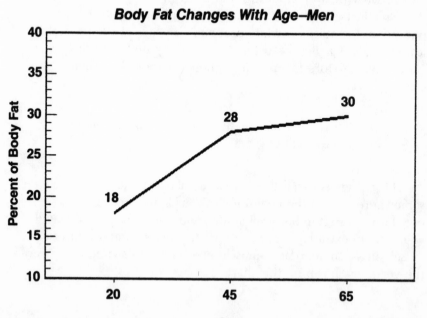

Body Fat Changes With Age–Men

The Incredible Shrinking Woman

In recent years, no disease has gotten more notice than osteo-porosis. Few people realize that this is not just a disease of bones that break, but also of *bones that actually shrink.*

By the time you are sixty-five, your body is only about half as efficient as it once was in absorbing mineral nutrients from foods. Instead of your body taking minerals like calcium, magnesium and potassium from your food, it borrows them from your bones. The bones weaken, losing, on average, 25 percent of their density.

This bone loss can take a significant toll on your height. For most people, the average length of the vertebral column is rela-tively constant—about 24 inches for women and 27 inches for men. That means, if you subtract the height of the leg bones, we are rather similar in height.

TALLNESS TEST

The next time you find yourself in a group of people of different height, observe carefully what happens as you sit down. When you sit, you are all more or less eye to eye, even though you may have to look up or down at them when you stand up. The differences in people's height are due mostly to the length of the leg bones.

As your body borrows minerals stored in the spinal vertebrae, those bones actually begin to collapse and compact, falling in on themselves. As your spinal column shrinks, you gradually lose the 24 inches or 27 inches of spine length you once had, and you become a "little old lady" or a "little old man."

The average American man can expect to lose up to 2¾ inches in height between the ages of 25 and 70; women, a less drastic 1⅞ inches. Sometimes, the loss is not so gradual: The collapse of just one of the vertebrae in the middle of the back can remove as much as 1⅛ inches of height.

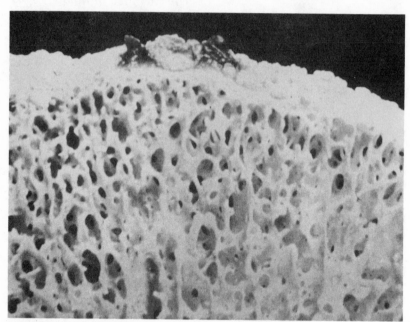

Normal mineral-rich bone

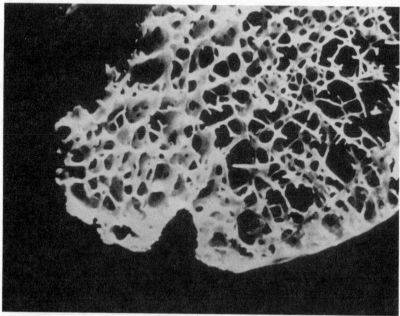

Mineral-depleted osteoporotic bone

Over the years, you can expect something like this:

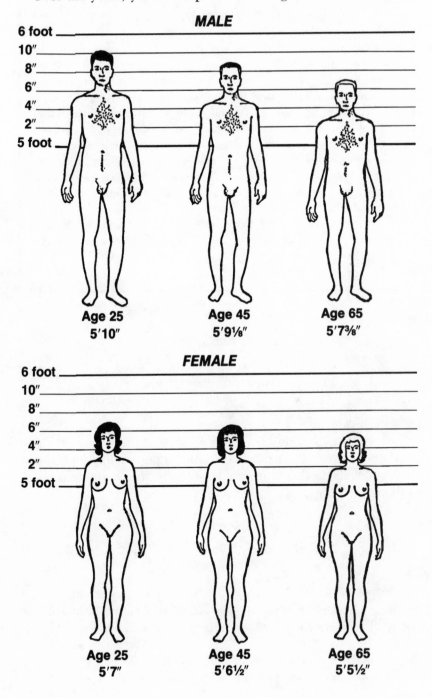

MALE

6 foot
10"
8"
6"
4"
2"
5 foot

Age 25
5'10"

Age 45
5'9⅛"

Age 65
5'7⅜"

FEMALE

6 foot
10"
8"
6"
4"
2"
5 foot

Age 25
5'7"

Age 45
5'6½"

Age 65
5'5½"

OUT OF ARM'S WAY . . .

Even your arms shrink as you age. Your arm span, measured from fingertip to fingertip with your arms outstretched, will be one-half less at age sixty-five than it is today. But through an interesting biological optical illusion, they appear to lengthen with age. The reason? Your arms shrink far less than your spine, so that as they hang next to your body, they will appear relatively longer.

The changes go all the way to your fingertips. Right now, if you are twenty years old, your nails take an average of one third less time to grow out than they will at age sixty. After another decade of getting older, by age seventy, they will grow less than half as fast as they do now.

But if you're worried that every part of you will shrink with age, don't—your feet, at least, actually become longer and enlarge as you age.

Face to Face with Age

At age 50, every man has the face he deserves.
—GEORGE ORWELL

Orwell was talking about the obvious, outward changes that are most noticeable in the face. Rather than reading all the biological details, in this case, you'll see the picture opposite is worth a thousand words:

Hair Today, Gone Tomorrow?

Not necessarily. It is true that hair undergoes major changes with age because it is one of the fastest-replicating tissues of the body. There are three primary changes you can expect:

—For both men and women, the hair becomes much finer. Each strand loses about one fifth of its thickness.

Facial Changes With Age

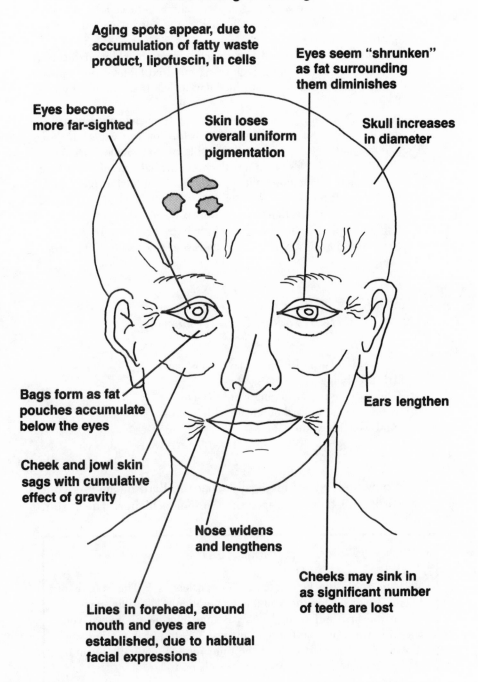

Aging spots appear, due to accumulation of fatty waste product, lipofuscin, in cells

Eyes seem "shrunken" as fat surrounding them diminishes

Eyes become more far-sighted

Skin loses overall uniform pigmentation

Skull increases in diameter

Bags form as fat pouches accumulate below the eyes

Ears lengthen

Cheek and jowl skin sags with cumulative effect of gravity

Nose widens and lengthens

Cheeks may sink in as significant number of teeth are lost

Lines in forehead, around mouth and eyes are established, due to habitual facial expressions

—Hair color comes from the pigment contained in each hair shaft. As you age, the coarse, pigmented hair is replaced by nonpigmented strands—and when you look in the mirror, you find more (gasp!) gray hairs.

—The density of individual hair follicles—how thickly your head is "forested"—drops from a high of six hundred follicles per square centimeter on your thirtieth birthday to half that number by age fifty.

—If you are a *man*, your hair will probably change its pattern of distribution, even if you do not go bald. You can expect to lose hair around your temples, the result of your male hormones. Whether you will also manifest the creeping hair loss of a receding hairline and a widening bald area on the crown of your pate, well, that depends on your genes.

—If you are a *woman*, there is a one-in-six chance that you will have lost most of your body and pubic hair by age sixty (unless you come from Japanese stock, in which case it is virtually 100 percent likely).

Hear Today, Gone Tomorrow?

. . . One man in his time plays many parts,
His acts being seven ages.
The sixth age . . . his big manly voice,
turning again toward childish treble, pipes
And whistles in his sound.
　　　　　　　　—*As You Like It,* Act II, scene vii

We now understand medically what the Bard meant. As your vocal cords pull taut with age, they resonate higher. The result:

"HUM" TEST

Hum softly the first notes of "Greensleeves" ("The Sounds of Silence" will do for the younger generation). The difference between the first and second notes is the difference between your speaking voice now and at age seventy. Or, to put it another way, if at seventy you start to hum the tune you will naturally begin on the same pitch that the second note falls on today.

Your speaking voice—in both men and women—rises about twenty-five cycles per second. To get an idea of how your speaking voice will rise, try the "hum" test.

More Than Skin Deep . . .

Perhaps the most profound changes happen where you can't see or hear them, deep within your cellular and organ systems. In virtually every niche and cranny of your body, aging means the power and strength of your organs and cells are gradual waning.

Losing Our Immunity?

Aging is the progressive accumulation of changes with time . . . associated with or responsible for the ever-increasing susceptibility to disease and death which accompanies old age.
    —Dr. Denham Harman, "The Aging Process," *Proceedings of the National Academy of Science,* November 1978.

The vulnerability he speaks of is intimately linked to the immune system. During your twenties and thirties, and particularly after age forty or so, your immune system begins to wane in several ways:

—Certain types of immune sentries—T cells, B cells, and neutrophils—become less efficient at protecting you from bacteria, viruses, and cancer.

—By age seventy, your immune system has lost 80 percent to 90 percent of the vigor and germ-fighting reserve it had when you were fifteen.

—Your body becomes less vigilant about fighting off threats to your health, leaving you more vulnerable to infections and cancer.

—Your immune troops become careless and imprecise, failing to distinguish adequately between enemy targets and friendly targets they should leave alone. When this happens, in what doctors call an "autoimmune response" ("auto" means "self"), your body starts to fight itself, even your most vital organs. When the armies that Nature gave you to defend your body turn mutinous, you pay a steep price.

When immune cells attack . . .	You get . . .
Joint linings	Rheumatoid arthritis
Pancreas cells	Diabetes
Nerve fibers	Multiple sclerosis
Stomach lining	Pernicious anemia
Liver	Chronic active hepatitis
Thyroid gland	Graves' disease

An aging immune system, then, is one that has grown both weak and careless.

Plumbing Problems

You can expect your urinary system to lose fully one half its efficiency between age thirty and age eighty. That means your kidneys filter only half as much blood waste per hour. At the same time, the walls of your bladder change, and its capacity diminishes. The result? Rest-room stops become more and more frequent—and urgent.

The body's electrical system, the nerves, also show signs of wear. Your overall muscle coordination and reflexes drop by one third to one quarter. Some of that is due to the speed of electrical nerve signals along the body, which slows down a few percent each decade. By your midsixties, those signals are traveling about 15 percent slower than they used to.

Are You All Wet?

Even your body's cells themselves change. For instance, do you believe that the body's cells become more or less moist with age? The answer may seem obvious: They actually lose moisture with each passing year, dropping from 42 percent to 33 percent of your body's composition from age twenty-five to seventy-five.

Neuro-muscular Changes With Age

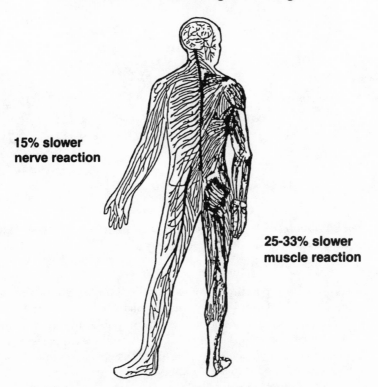

**15% slower
nerve reaction**

**25-33% slower
muscle reaction**

This dryness may be part of what accounts for the general sensation of losing the suppleness and silkiness of youth.

There is a very important practical consideration you should know about. As you age, you need to take smaller drug doses to get the same effect. Partly that is due to the fact that your liver and kidneys perform less efficiently. But we know now that part is also due to the greater concentration of drugs in your cells, which in older adults are less diluted by cellular fluids.

Oxygen Changes

One of the most profound changes comes in how your body processes oxygen. Oxygen, of course, is the fuel that stokes your cellular energy furnaces. As the years pass, the oxygen processing mechanism changes in two main ways:

Oxygen Processing Losses With Age

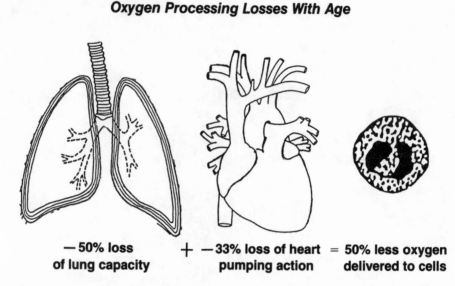

— 50% loss of lung capacity	+ — 33% loss of heart pumping action	= 50% less oxygen delivered to cells

—Your lung capacity drops from six to three quarts of air with each breath. Right there, less oxygen is available to your bloodstream.

—Then, the average American heart loses up to a third of its pumping capacity, due to the damage caused by disease processes that appear with increasing age. The pumping rate may drop from a high of almost four quarts a minute at age twenty-five to only two and a half quarts at age sixty-five.

This adds up to a significant double whammy: By retirement age, your cells may be getting just half the oxygen they were getting when you graduated college. Small wonder every set of stairs seems to get steeper!

Lowering the Energy Throttle

The common perception of "losing energy" with age reflects a profound biologic truth. Your *basal metabolism*—the rate at which your body burns fuel—drops almost 3 percent every decade. By age seventy, it has tapered off by about one fifth from its peak when you were young. In effect, your body's engines throttle themselves down, bit by inevitable bit.

Time for "Young Blood"?

You probably don't think of your blood as a part of your body that ages particularly, but it does. All of your blood cells are constantly being replaced, and of the approximately twenty-odd trillion blood cells in your body right now, none is older than about four months. However, the real shift comes in the overall chemical profile of the four quarts (men, make that six) of red stuff in your arteries.

Reading Your Own "Blood Age Print"

As you age, the combination of chemicals in your blood changes significantly. If you are a healthy thirty-four-year-old, how your blood profile looks today has little in common with how it will look at age sixty. That means the blood system carries its own rough "age print" which a blood expert (hematologist) can "read" to get a rough idea of how far along you are in the aging process. To cite just four vital measures:

—Blood chemicals, like the hormone renin aldosterone and the blood component albumin, drop as we age. Others, like glucose, uric acid, and the abnormal protein called rheumatoid factor, rise.
—Your blood pressure creeps up over the years, so that what would be a worrisome elevation in a twenty-five-year-old is just about average for his or her mother. Most of us can expect our overall blood pressure to increase about 15 percent between the ages of thirty and sixty-five.
—Likewise, you can expect your cholesterol to rise—for a while. A level of 220 would be of some concern in a twenty-five-year-old, but just about normal at age fifty. But then, after about age fifty-five, it starts inching its way back down again.
—Your blood level of abnormal proteins increases. One of these proteins, rheumatoid factor, is implicated in arthritic inflammation of the joints.

Come to Your Senses . . .

[The] last scene of all . . .
Sans teeth, sans eyes, sans taste, sans everything.
—*As You Like It*, Act II, scene vii

It is a common view that our older years should be a time to "stop and smell the roses," but unfortunately Nature has built in an obstacle. Experiments suggest that the sense of smell declines significantly with age, particularly for men.

Happily, though, Nature does not rob you of all senses equally. Shakespeare notwithstanding, the sense of taste is very little affected directly by age.

TAKE THE TONGUE TEST

Look at your tongue in the mirror, you will see that it is covered with small bumps, or *papillae*. If you looked at these bumps under a microscope, you would see that each contains a total of between two thousand and nine thousand taste buds—the nerve endings that register sweet, sour, salt, and bitter, and tell you the difference between lime sherbet, fresh peaches, and chopped liver.

Starting at age fifty, the taste buds become less able to regenerate. Within about twenty years, perhaps 70 percent have died off, leaving a scanty seventy-five taste buds on each papilla.

We become less sensitive to the four basic tastes after age fifty. Happily, this loss doesn't lead to a corresponding two-thirds drop in your tasting enjoyment, because Nature has built in redundancy to the human body. If you do lose some sense of taste with age, it is most likely due to some other reason—drugs, sickness, even changes in nerve-transmitter chemicals in the brain.

Ah yes, the brain. Most of us think of the brain as one of the most vulnerable organs to the ravages of age. From a biological perspective, that is accurate: Your brain shrinks, losing about 10

Loss of Taste Buds With Age

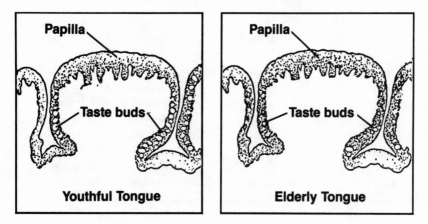

percent of its sixteen billion nerve cells by age seventy, and about 40 percent of its weight.

It is a rough-and-ready rule of thumb that if aging is left to its own course you can count on it robbing your body of about 1 percent of its overall functional capacity each year after about age 35. Notice that I said "left to its own course"—after all, you wouldn't be reading this book if you were planning to leave aging to its own course!

Your Body's Functional Capacity

> There is a wicked inclination in most people to suppose an old man decayed in his intellects. If a young or middle-aged man, when leaving a company, does not recollect where he laid his hat, it is nothing; but let the same inattention be discovered in an old man and people shrug and say, "His memory is going."
>
> —SAMUEL JOHNSON

Samuel Johnson's wise observation is echoed by the newest brain research. Despite physical losses, it just isn't true that we face an inevitable loss of our thinking and brainpower as we age,

ADD IT ALL UP AND WHAT DO YOU GET?

Brain weight	decreases 40% by age 70
Number of nerve trunk fibers	decreases 37% by age 70
Blood flow to brain	decreases 20% by age 70
Speed of blood equilibrium mechanism	decreases 83% by age 70
Basal metabolic rate	decreases 20% by age 70
Kidney filtration rate	decreases 50% by age 70
Body water content	decreases 15% by age 70
Resting heart output	decreases 30% by age 70
Handgrip strength	decreases 45% by age 70
Oxygen uptake while exercising	decreases 60% by age 70
Lung volume during exercise	decreases 47% by age 70

and it most certainly doesn't have to happen to you. Consider recent research findings:

—"Despite the common belief, thinking can actually improve with age."—New York Hospital–Cornell Medical Center.

—"In every age group, even among the oldest, individuals were found whose performance on mental tasks did not decline with age, but was indistinguishable from that of younger adults."—*Handbook of the Biology of Aging,* 1985.

—"At all ages the majority of people maintain their levels of intellectual competence—or actually improve—as they grow older."—National Institute on Aging.

My medical training showed me firsthand just how one can keep intellectual abilities sharp into the most advanced age. I will never forget the staggering intellect of one of my medical professors, a man who is now on the near side of eighty. He was held in awe for his razor-sharp intellect and total recall, which were terribly intimidating to my cadre of green medical students. Woe to the poor young intern who made the mistake of supposing that Dr. Weinstein had lost any of his faculties!

Aging Overview

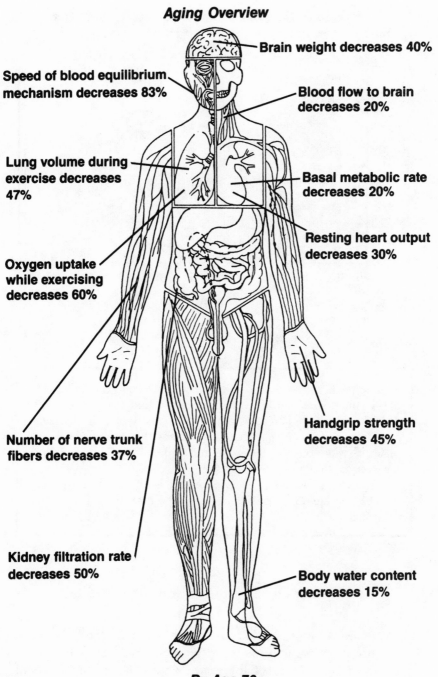

Brain weight decreases 40%

Speed of blood equilibrium mechanism decreases 83%

Blood flow to brain decreases 20%

Lung volume during exercise decreases 47%

Basal metabolic rate decreases 20%

Resting heart output decreases 30%

Oxygen uptake while exercising decreases 60%

Number of nerve trunk fibers decreases 37%

Handgrip strength decreases 45%

Kidney filtration rate decreases 50%

Body water content decreases 15%

By Age 70

Change of Overall Functional Capacity with Age

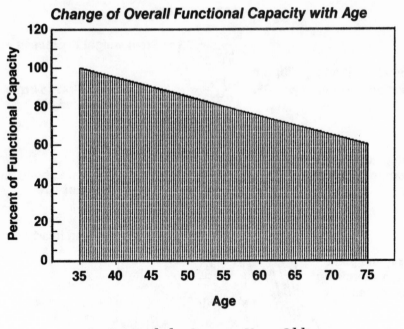

Sex and the Seventy-Year-Old

One other bit of good news: Obviously, a woman's hormonal profile changes dramatically with menopause, and it has long been thought that men's hormones showed a similar waning in their later years. Happily, current research indicates that the levels of the male sex hormones testosterone and androgen in older men remain equal to those of their sons, even grandsons.

The best part of this prescription is that the levels of sex hormones stay highest among those men who have the highest level of sexual activity.

The Anti-aging Motto: Use It or Lose It

We now understand that to a great extent the body operates on a "use it or lose it" principle. That is true of heart, mind, and muscles. That means that there are ways to make sure you will be as sharp, vital, and alive in thirty years as you are right now.

If there is one youth secret that runs through all the research on growth and aging, and throughout this book, it is summed up in those five words—use it or lose it. You possess the keys to staying young and vital—if you choose to use them.

Let's Get Personal

Let's bring this down to a very personal level and look at how these changes will touch *your* life (how much more personal can you get than inside your own body?). You will dust off your crystal ball and peer into the decades ahead.

Using some basic medical tools, you can in effect project your medical future with some educated guesses about what your body will look, act, and feel like as you age.

Dear Old Mom and Dad—Your Aging Blueprint

You already own the simplest tool to give you a hint about your medical future—the family photo album. Take a look at a picture of your parents or grandparents when they were your age. Look at their hairlines, their body shape, their weight distribution, their faces—then and now. Do you see something of yourself in them (or, more accurately, vice-versa)?

Now compare earlier photographs of them with later ones. In a very real way, the differences your parents have manifested over two decades are a blueprint for the changes you can reasonably expect to experience as you grow older.

—Did your mother develop the bent-over "dowager's hump" that signals osteoporosis?
—Did your father's joints swell with rheumatoid arthritis?
—Did they lose their looks and vitality, or stay hale and hearty until relatively late in life?

There is a solid scientific reason for this exercise. Your parents, after all, are practically your closest genetic match—they just have a twenty- or thirty-year jump on you in how long they've aged, and are the best living examples of how your basic gene set is likely to age.

Aging Forecaster

The second method is more scientific, based on data gathered in examining thousands of people. It takes into account certain average changes that come with age. These data are based on a statistical golden mean, and there is no guarantee that you will age exactly the same way, but it certainly gives you a general idea about what the decades ahead may hold for you.

Fill in as many of the answers in the lefthand column as you can. Then follow the instructions in the middle column, and be-

Your Personal Aging Forecaster

Your current:	Factor in these biological changes:	Personal prediction at age 70:
Weight	Men: Subtract 7% Women: Add 4%	
Height	Men: subtract 2½" Women: subtract 1¾"	
Number of teeth: _____ (32, if none are lost yet)	Subtract 1 tooth per decade	
Blood pressure	Men: add 20/10 Women: add 30/10	
Overall functional capacity, start with 100% at age 25	Subtract 10% for each decade	
Body temperature	Subtract 1.5 degrees	
Cholesterol	Men add 40 points Women add 50 points	

hold! the righthand column will give you a reasonable extrapolation of where you might find yourself a few years from now.

Certain aspects affecting your health are such important variables that they merit a more in-depth, and more precise, prediction.

BLOOD PRESSURE PREDICTOR

Biostatistics let us create a more accurate model to predict possible changes in your blood pressure over the coming years. To predict your possible blood pressure at a given age, use the charts on page 66.

1. Find that age along the line at the bottom of the first chart.
2. Looking at the correct line for your gender, read straight across to the vertical line to find a number. That number represents the top number (systolic) of your blood pressure reading.
3. Do the same on the second chart. That number represents the bottom number (diastolic) of your blood pressure reading.
4. Now, for your final result:

Number from
top chart

At age _____ my blood pressure may be: _____

Number from
bottom chart

You can customize this for yourself even more accurately if you know your current blood pressure.

5. If you know your current blood pressure, write numbers here:__

6. Next, find the average blood pressure for your age category in the table below:

Age	Average Male Blood Pressure	Average Female Blood Pressure
18–24	124/76	111/70
25–34	125/79	112/73
35–44	126/82	119/78
45–54	131/85	129/82

Systolic Blood Pressure Changes With Age

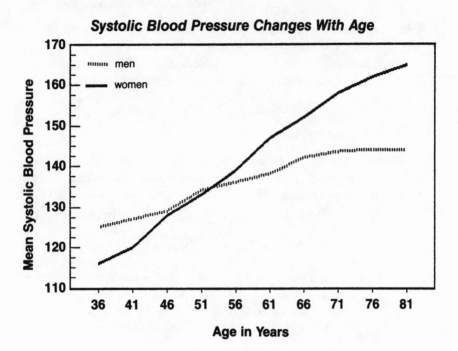

Diastolic Blood Pressure Changes With Age

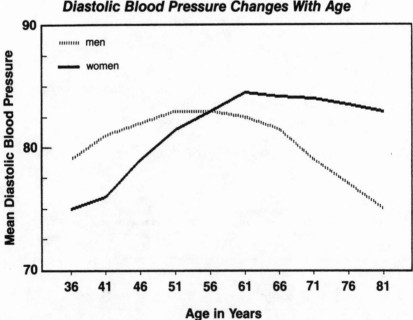

7. Subtract the blood pressure number shown in the table from your current blood pressure and write the difference here:_____ (Don't worry if it's negative—it just means you have a lower-than-average blood pressure profile.)
8. Add the number from step 7 and the number from step 4 here for your personalized prediction:_____.

GUESS YOUR WEIGHT

Unlike getting on the scales down at the local drugstore, this is done with the help of medical epidemiology. Use the chart on page 68.

YOUR CHOLESTEROL COMPUTER

If your doctor has told you what your cholesterol level is, you can proceed with this test.

1. Find your age on the chart below, depending on your gender.
2. If your current cholesterol level is approximately equal to that

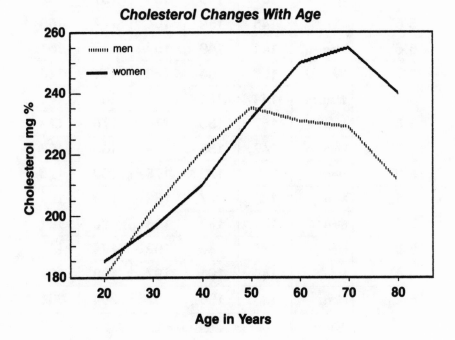

Cholesterol Changes With Age

Ideal Weight Chart

YOUR HEIGHT		AGE				
		18-24	25-34	35-44	45-54	55-64
4'10"	Women	114	123	133	132	135
4'11"	Women	118	126	136	136	138
5'0"	Women	121	130	139	139	142
5'1"	Women	124	133	141	143	145
5'2"	Men	130	139	146	148	147
5'2"	Women	128	136	144	146	148
5'3"	Men	135	145	149	154	151
5'3"	Women	131	139	146	150	151
5'4"	Men	139	151	155	158	156
5'4"	Women	134	142	149	153	154
5'5"	Men	143	155	159	163	160
5'5"	Women	137	146	151	157	157
5'6"	Men	148	159	164	167	165
5'6"	Women	141	149	154	160	161
5'7"	Men	152	164	169	171	170
5'7"	Women	144	152	156	164	164
5'8"	Men	157	168	174	176	174
5'8"	Women	147	155	159	168	167
5'9"	Men	162	173	178	180	178
5'10"	Men	166	177	183	185	183
5'11"	Men	171	182	188	190	187
6'0"	Men	175	186	192	194	192
6'1"	Men	180	191	197	198	197
6'2"	Men	185	196	202	204	201

Calculated from: U.S. Center for Health Statistics, North American Association Study of Obesity.

indicated for your age and gender, you can follow this curve up to get a rough average prediction of your cholesterol later in life.

3. If your current cholesterol level differs widely from that shown in the chart, determine the difference. (For example, a thirty-year-old woman should have a level of no more than 190. If yours is 205, the difference is 15 points.)

4. Add the point difference from step 3 to the age-adjusted value you found in step 2. This gives an approximate range that you might hit at that age—providing you don't make changes in your diet, exercise, or medications.

You may want to copy down these predictive results and file them away. Twenty weeks from now, when you have had a chance to incorporate many of the basic longevity steps outlined in this book into your life, you might want to consult these results. If you do, I think you may find a pleasant surprise: Thanks to this book, and the changes you have made in your life, you will have improved your score on these variables. But more important than your test score is how you feel, look, and act. Because in those twenty weeks you will have started making yourself biologically younger than your present chronological age.

So next time you hear someone say, "You're not getting any younger," remember your twenty-two longevity steps and smile— because you'll know better.

4
How Old Are You, Really?

"This is it. This is what fifty looks like."
—Gloria Steinem, on being told how young she looked on her fiftieth birthday.

IF YOU ARE to commit to making yourself younger, you have to know where to start—to know how old your body systems are right now. That seems easy—you know how old you are, right? Medically speaking, that isn't necessarily accurate.

A range of biological factors makes the body's real biological age—where its physical systems fall along the continuum from birth to death—only loosely related to the number of years since birth. From your body's perspective, your age is an absolutely relative, approximate measure. You have surely heard a "youthful" seventy-year-old say of a young person that he is "old beyond his years," or have watched a friend age quickly in a few months' time. In each of those instances, you have picked up on a series of subtle—and not-so-subtle—clues about the energy, vitality, mental acuity, general fitness, and sharpness of these people's senses and reflexes, as well as a broad range of different elements about their biological, social, and psychological functioning.

Too, not all parts of your body age at the same rate. You may have a heart that functions at a level "younger" than the age shown on your driver's license, thanks to careful diet and exercise. Yet your skin, liver, or other organs may function like the organs of someone much older because of genetic weakness or stresses they have endured.

71

Reckoning how the body's systems work is what I do with my patients, and what your own family doctor does during your physical. As your physician checks out your heart and lungs, bones and mobility, blood pressure and lab results, she or he is in effect assessing how you are doing relative to others of the same approximate age. It is when you fall outside the range of age-adjusted values that you are diagnosed with some problem.

In this chapter, you will do much the same thing, assessing your body's relative biological age—what I call your "Youth Quotient."

Your Personal "Youth Quotient" Assessment

YOUR PHYSIOLOGY

1. Is your blood pressure: _____

    A. In the range of 120/80–140/90 (1)
    B. Above 140/90 (10)
    C. Above 95/60 but below 120/80 (−10)
    D. Less than 95/60 (10)

2. Is your blood cholesterol level: _____

    A. More than 260 (15)
    B. Between 230 and 260 (10)
    C. Between 180 and 220 (1)
    D. Between 140 and 180 (−10)
    E. Below 140 (−5)

3. Is your resting pulse: _____

    A. Less than 60 beats per minute (−10)
    B. 60–70 beats per minute (1)
    C. 70–90 beats per minute (10)
    D. More than 90 beats per minute (15)

4. Has your doctor ever told you that you are anemic?   _____

    A. Yes (10)
    B. No (1)

5. Are you: ____

  A. 20% or more above desired weight (10)
  B. 5%–20% overweight (5)
  C. About right for your height (1)
  D. 5–20% underweight (5)
  E. 20% or more under (8)

6. Compared to this time last year, your weight: ____

  A. Is pretty much the same (1)
  B. Has risen or fallen, but you can control it with diet
     and exercise (5)
  C. Is rising or falling now, and is very hard to maintain (10)

FAMILY HISTORY

7. Do any family members have diabetes, hypertension, or
   heart disease?   ____

  A. No (1)
  B. Yes (10)

8. Has anyone in your family ever been diagnosed with cancer? ____

  A. No. (1)
  B. Yes (5)

9. Do others in your family have severe allergies?   ____

  A. No, not that I know of (1)
  B. Yes, mostly hay fever (3)
  C. Yes, significant allergies to foods or environment (5)

10. Do you have trouble breathing, shortness of breath?   ____

  A. No (1)
  B. Sometimes, but infrequently (5)
  C. This is a regular or common feeling (10)

11. Do you cough when you wake up in the morning?   ____

  A. Almost never, except when I have flu or a cold (1)
  B. Sometimes, but it passes quickly (5)
  C. This happens regularly (10)

IMMUNE FUNCTION

12. Do you frequently catch cold, flu, or other illnesses? ____

    A. Never—or very rarely (1)
    B. 2–4 times a year (5)
    C. More than 4 times a year (10)

13. When you get sick, how long does it usually take to recover fully? ____

    A. 3–4 days (1)
    B. About 10 days (5)
    C. I haven't felt really well for a very long time (10)
    D. Can't remember the last time I was sick (−10)

14. Do you have a history of chronic illness? ____

    A. No (−10)
    B. Yes, but for less than 5 years (5)
    C. Yes, for 5 or more years (10)

15. When you get a cut or bruise, does it heal quickly? ____

    A. Yes, it usually heals completely in a few days (1)
    B. I have noticed that I heal more slowly than I used to (5)
    C. Bruises stay a long time; cuts leave a visible mark (10)

16. Your overall health is: ____

    A. Excellent—I am very satisfied (1)
    B. Usually all right, but could be better (5)
    C. Fair to poor—I wish it were better (10)

SPECIFIC SYMPTOMS

17. Have you noticed any problems with walking, balance, or coordination? ____

    A. No (1)
    B. Yes, ongoing minor problems (5)
    C. Yes, they significantly impair my movement (10)

18. How is your skin?   ____

    A. Smooth and supple, not scaly or irritated (1)
    B. Rough, cracked, dry in some months.
       Occasional problem patches (5)
    C. Chronically dry, itchy, flaky, or irritated (10)

19. Do you have headaches?   ____

    A. A few times a year, or less (1)
    B. Often, but they go away quickly (5)
    C. Often, and they are painful and debilitating (10)

20. Do you experience leg or arm muscle cramps?   ____

    A. No, almost never (1)
    B. Occasionally—sometimes when I am sleeping (5)
    C. Yes, frequently, especially when I walk or exercise (10)

21. Do you have arthritis, joint pain, or pain in your feet and
    hands?   ____

    A. Only rarely (1)
    B. My joints sometimes seem stiff; I notice pain in my
       hands and feet more (5)
    C. Pain in joints and extremities has really limited my
       mobility or actions (10)

22. Do you have pain in your back, especially down low?   ____

    A. Only rarely, and it goes away (1)
    B. Twinges, but not debilitating (5)
    C. It is a constant feeling, and affects my mobility, actions,
       or mood (10)

23. Do your extremities ever feel cold, numb, or tingly?   ____

    A. No, I do not experience those feelings (1)
    B. They happen sometimes, but not regularly (5)
    C. Yes, I have noticed those sensations regularly (10)

24. Do you get diarrhea, constipation, or digestion problems? ____

    A. No, or only when I am ill or have eaten the wrong
       foods (1)
    B. Yes, but the problems are more irritating than serious (5)
    C. These are frequent problems; I watch carefully what I
       eat (10)

EXERCISE

25. When was the last time you did any strenuous exercise? ____

    A. Within the last 5 days (−10)
    B. Only within the last month (1)
    C. Longer than a month (10)

26. Do you get out of breath? ____

    A. When I do strenuous aerobic exercise for more than a few minutes (−10)
    B. Whenever I exercise or have a short exertion like running for a bus or playing with a child for a little while (5)
    C. When I climb stairs or carry parcels (10)

27. Do your legs cramp when you walk more than a few minutes? ____

    A. As a regular occurrence (10)
    B. Sometimes, but rarely (5)
    C. No (1)

28. Have you had any broken bones in the last year? ____

    A. No (1)
    B. Yes, one incident (5)
    C. Two or more separate times (10)

29. Your general energy level is: ____

    A. Variable—some days I feel fine, but mostly I could use more energy (5)
    B. Great—I have lots of energy (1)
    C. Consistently sluggish. I often want to sleep. When I do, I often don't awake refreshed (10)

NUTRITION AND DIET

30. When it comes to fiber in your food, you: ____

    A. Consciously eat raw vegetables and fruits, grains, and legumes (−10)
    B. Usually eat at least a salad once a day, whole grains or equivalent (1)

C. Eat mostly frozen or canned vegetables (5)

D. I don't like vegetables or grains (10)

31. Does *most* of your protein come from: _____

    A. Veal, white-meat chicken (5)
    B. Vegetable sources (nuts, grains, or legumes) or fish (−5)
    C. Red meat (10)

32. How often do you eat fried foods, butter, or other choles-
    terol-containing foods?   _____

    A. More than once a day (10)
    B. About once a day (5)
    C. Less than once a day (−5)

33. Do you eat cruciferous vegetables (cauliflower, broccoli,
    Brussels sprouts)?   _____

    A. At least once a week, fresh (−5)
    B. No more than occasionally (5)
    C. Hardly ever or never (10)

34. What about calcium?   _____

    A. I know the calcium content of foods and make an effort to
       eat calcium-rich foods (−5)
    B. I take calcium supplements (1)
    C. I don't make any special effort (10)

35. Do you eat more: _____

    A. Simple carbohydrates (candy, sweets, jelly, desserts) (10)
    B. Complex carbohydrates (pasta, bread, grains) (−5)

36. Do you salt your food: _____

    A. Heavily (10)
    B. Lightly (5)
    C. Not at all (1)

37. Have you noticed allergies to any food or drink?   _____

    A. No, nothing obvious (1)
    B. Yes, to 1 or 2 specific items (5)
    C. Yes, to 3 or more food or drink items (10)

LIFE-STYLE AND HABITS

38. Do you drink alcohol? ____

    A. More than 2 drinks per day (10)
    B. 2 drinks per day (3)
    C. Occasionally, less than 2 drinks daily (−5)
    D. No (−10)

39. Do you always wear seat belts? ____

    A. Yes (1)
    B. No (10)

40. Do you smoke cigars, pipes, or cigarettes? ____

    A. Yes (10)
    B. No (−10)

41. Do you breathe others' smoke at home or at work? ____

    A. Yes (10)
    B. No (1)

42. If you are light-skinned, do you take measures to protect your skin from the sun? ____

    A. Yes, I stay out of the sun or remain thoroughly covered (1)
    B. Yes, I wear sunscreen (5)
    C. No, I like looking tanned and healthy (10)

43. Which best describes your sleeping habits? ____

    A. I usually get 6–8 hours of sleep a night; I awaken refreshed (1)
    B. I don't always get enough sleep, but catch up on weekends (5)
    C. I have problems falling asleep, wake through the night, have trouble waking in the morning, or don't feel rested (10)

44. When it comes to worrying: ____

    A. Once I make up my mind, I don't look back. Fretting is not my style. I leave problems at work (1)
    B. Like most people, I have a lot on my mind sometimes, but not usually (5)

C. I often worry about things that haven't happened yet.
I replay what I should have said or done in situations (10)

45. How many prescription drugs do you take?   ____

    A. None, have never taken them regularly (1)
    B. 1–3 types of drugs now or in the last year (5)
    C. At least 4 types now or in the last year (10)

EMOTIONAL STATUS

46. About your work life and career choice: ____

    A. I really enjoy my job and the challenge it brings me (1)
    B. I am generally satisfied, but sometimes it gives me
       real problems (5)
    C. My job is a chore, I wish I were somewhere else (10)

47. Is there someone in your life you trust absolutely and can
    tell your deepest secrets to?   ____

    A. Yes, my mate or best friend (−10)
    B. Usually, but I don't often bother people with my
       problems (5)
    C. There is no one in my life I can confide in right now,
       I tend to be a loner (10)

48. In life: ____

    A. I am quite independent in making decisions that affect
       me (1)
    B. Much of what I do depends on my mate, boss, family,
       or others. Sometimes I don't feel in control (5)
    C. My life is very constrained by others (10)

49. Does your life allow you to really enjoy your friends and
    hobbies?   ____

    A. Yes, I am pretty happy with my balanced life-style (−5)
    B. My time is mostly dedicated to obligations and duties (5)
    C. I can't remember the last time I really had great fun (10)

50. Right now, you would describe your emotional state as: ____

    A. Pretty upbeat and stable, all things considered (1)
    B. It varies, but I don't get too down or stay that way (5)
    C. My life feels pretty bleak and out of control (10)

51. Your sexual relations are: ____

    A. Satisfying and positive (1)
    B. Some areas definitely need help (5)
    C. A significant issue—I have no satisfying sexual outlet (10)

52. Choose the phrase that best describes you: ____

    A. Calm, even-tempered and generally happy. Friends
       comment on it (1)
    B. A "hard worker" with high standards at work, school,
       in relationships. Trying to keep everything under
       control, I don't always succeed (5)
    C. I am under heavy stress. I am quick to anger (10)

53. Your relations with others tend to be: ____

    A. Satisfying, with clear lines of communication (1)
    B. A strain. I often feel like I can't connect (5)
    C. Often short-lived and marked by disputes (10)

54. When you look in a mirror, you feel: ____

    A. I look good for someone my age, as well as I feel (-5)
    B. I could look better with some work on diet, exercise,
       etc. (1)
    C. To look good is a major, difficult effort (10)

SCORING:

                    Total score for your biological age: ____

1. Write your chronological age here: ____
2. Look up your total score to find your biological age and your
   Youth Preservation Level: ____

Pay Special Attention to Your Youth Preservation Level

That letter is your key to the Youth Preservation steps you
will be making in every chapter from now on. If you are in Level
A, you will have a different regime than if you are in Level D
throughout this book. You need to know your Youth Preservation
Level in order to tailor the Youth Preservation steps to you.

Score	Your Biological Age	Youth Preservation Level
−82 to 43	Subtract 5 Years from Chronological Age	A
43 to 170	Subtract 2 years from Chronological Age	B
170 to 296	Keep Chronological Age Unchanged	C
296 to 423	Add 2 Years to Chronological Age	D
423 to 550	Add 5 Years to Chronological Age	E

Grand total for Your Biological Age: _____

If you don't like what you see right now, as you add up the grand total, remember: The farther behind you are, the greater your potential to make tremendous, positive changes in your health and life expectancy. You may want to take this quiz again after you have made the life-style changes in the chapters that follow. I guarantee that you will score "younger"—because biologically your body's processes will actually *be* younger.

5

Keeping the Outer You Looking Young

THE FIRST PLACE to start making yourself younger is where it is most obvious—with the body that greets you in the mirror and which everybody sees. This chapter focuses on that outer you, your skin and face. It gives you six easy steps that you can do, right now, to make yourself look younger and regain the glow of youthful, radiant skin. Follow these steps, and in ten weeks from now you will start to see results. By the time you are twenty weeks into the program, I expect you will see a significant improvement in your skin's health and appearance.

But first, let's settle one thing once and for all. Many of my patients, when they first consult me for ways to make themselves look more youthful, confide this to me as though it were a dirty little secret. They think the idea of taking care of themselves is vain somehow. I disagree. Our society places an obsessive value on youth and vitality. Much of our power as individuals, and our self-worth, is intimately related to how youthful we, and others, feel we look. Appearance is the face you present to the world and, as such, it is very important. Outward appearances are far more than empty vanity.

Happily, mainstream medicine is now coming to agree. Note this editorial in the *Journal of the American Medical Association:*

It is increasingly apparent that appearance, certainly including cutaneous appearance, contributes to society's evaluation of an individual's competence and to that individual's sense of self-worth and well-being. . . . The prospect of [an] effective anti-aging product for the skin may have direct medical benefit beyond its effect on premalignant lesions.—*JAMA*, 1/22/88, Vol. 259, No. 4, p. 569

Translation: Experts realize that *looking as young as you feel is a vital part of being a vital person.*

The public has understood this fact longer than the doctors have. In the time it takes you to read this page, Americans will have spent $19,000 on skin preparations—a rate that adds up to a whopping $27 million every day! It's not just women; men, too, are finally starting to understand that looking their best makes them feel their best.

At the same time, scientists have found a fascinating relation between how old somebody looks to an observer and their scores on a battery of laboratory tests that measure aging throughout the body's systems. It seems that youthful-looking people have bodies that function biologically below their chronological age, and the reverse is true of people who look prematurely aged—independent of their chronological age. Clearly, inside and out, looking young is part of what it is to *be* young.

What's in Store for Your Skin?

Consider the difference between old and young skin (opposite).

As your skin ages, here's what happens biologically:

—You lose elasticity.
—You lose 10% to 20% of your skin's pigment cells each decade (that's why very old people seem to have such light, almost translucent skin).
—You lose 50 percent of the Langerhans cells, immune cells that protect against skin cancer.
—Your skin gets rougher and less evenly pigmented (age spots).
—Your skin turns from a rosy color to a more yellowish hue.

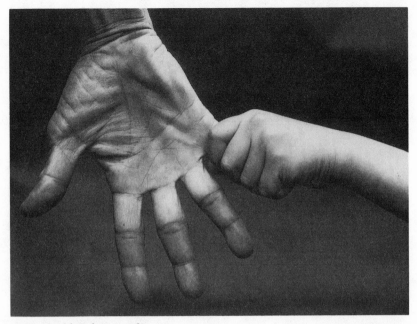

Compare old and young skin.

National Institute on Aging

Just a Pinch . . .

The Pinch Test is an approximate way to test your skin's age. Put your hand flat on a table, back side up. Pinch a fingerful of loose skin on the back of your hand between thumb and forefinger of your other hand, then let it go. Note how long it takes until the area you pinched has flattened out completely. That time suggests a reading of your skin's relative age.

That's a picture of what happens if Nature takes its course. Now let's see what you can do about it—the good news here. Today, there is an array of quite effective ways to keep your skin young and supple. Best of all, they are ways that work! Let's look at the six skin-care principles, combining nutrition, several new developments in skin products, and a few commonsense changes. With them, you can not only dramatically slow the rate of your skin's aging, but actually *reverse* some of the ravages that time has wrought.

Time for Pinch to Return to Normal

Women	Men	Skin Age
0 sec	0 sec	10–19
0 sec	0 sec	20–29
1 sec	<.5 sec	30–39
3 sec	1 sec	40–49
12 sec	4 sec	50–59
21 sec	20 sec	60–69
1 min	43 sec	Over 70

Step One: The Tretinoin "Miracle"

You have probably heard of last year's dermatologic superstar, topical tretinoin, or Retin-A. Just last year, the *Journal of the American Medical Association* caused an immense public stir when it published a study showing that this vitamin A-derived cream actually seems to reverse some of the changes caused by aging, renewing and rebuilding skin cells so the skin is less rough, mottled, and wrinkled. Where most creams merely hydrate your skin— that is, restore lost water and puff it up—Retin-A goes deeper into the dermal layers and actually stimulates new cell growth. The result? Your skin gains a new lease on life, actually filling in small creases and wrinkles, smoothing out rough spots. Since this discovery, Retin-A has been flying off pharmacists' shelves, and dermatologists have hardly been able to keep up with the demand.

The excitement is because Retin-A is the first product that can demonstrably, dependably make skin look younger. It smoothes out fine wrinkles, sun spots, and skin blemishes. It clearly promotes the growth of new, healthy skin, lifts the top surface of the skin away from deeper layers, and increases the rate of formation of new skin cells. The result is that Retin-A–treated skin is rejuvenated; creating not just new skin but more healthy, rosy, and fresh-looking skin. It is no miracle cure, surely, but one of the best tools to soften and lighten the patina of age that starts taking its toll on our faces after age thirty. I have seen Retin-A make positive changes in many patients after just several months.

You can expect it to:

—Help minor wrinkles, such as those around the nose and eyes
—Reduce blemishes, discoloration, or sun spots
—Help give your skin a better tone
—Make your skin somewhat softer and smoother
—Restore a more rosy glow to your skin

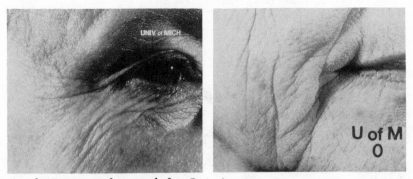

Facial appearance of woman before Retin-A

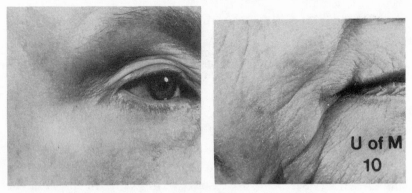

After ten months of Retin-A, smoother skin

John J. Vorhees, M.D.
University of Michigan Medical School

But don't expect a complete face-lift in a tube. Deep wrinkles and furrows will remain unchanged. And do be patient. After all, what Nature did in decades you can't expect to undo in weeks. You will probably require six months of daily applications to begin to appreciate fully the noticeable improvement in your skin's texture and luster.

ARE YOU A RETIN-A CANDIDATE?

Some people are ideal Retin-A candidates because of their skin type. Are you:

—Of Celtic origin (Irish, Scottish, English)?
—With blond or red hair?
—With fair skin?
—With blue eyes?
—One who spends any time in the sun?

If your answer to several of these questions is yes, congratulations: You are the ideal candidate to reverse the damages of skin aging by Retin-A. That doesn't mean other people won't be helped, too. It's just that they are most sensitive to the kind of sunlight damage that Retin-A works best on. But since almost all of us have some degree of photoaging, we, too, can be candidates for "saving face" with Retin-A.

PUTTING IT TO WORK IN YOUR OWN LIFE

If you are interested in Retin-A for you, the first step is to discuss it with a knowledgeable dermatologist. He or she will probably start you off with the 0.1 percent dosage concentration that is most widely used. Nine out of ten people have a reaction when they first use the cream—discomfort, peeling, or irritation. Don't worry—that is an expected and customary phase of your body's adaptation to the biological power of Retin-A.

Then, as you get used to the treatment, many doctors including Dr. Albert Kligman, professor emeritus of dermatology at the University of Pennsylvania, who discovered Retin-A's anti-aging properties, recommend increasing the dosage concentration to 0.2 percent or 0.5 percent after a period of time, if your skin can tolerate it.

To help make Retin-A available to everybody who could benefit from it, the makers of Retin-A have just announced that they will manufacture a special quarter-strength .025 percent version. This formulation should be available in your pharmacy by the time you read this. This means that many people with sensitive skin, who might have problems tolerating the full-strength 0.1 percent-formulation Retin-A, can still take advantage of its real wrinkle-smoothing benefits.

Retin-A is almost as easy to use as cold cream. Just spread a pea-sized dab of it each night on your face and neck. I usually start patients on an every-other-day regimen, to let their skin get used to the cream. If you tolerate it well, you can then slowly increase the frequency to once a day. If your skin gets irritated, ask your doctor for a lower concentration or use the cream every third day, until the redness goes away, then try returning to a more frequent schedule.

The latest research suggests that you should get the most significant cosmetic results in the first year and a half that you use Retin-A. At that point, the improvement seems to level off, and you can go on a less frequent maintenance regime that keeps the positive changes you have gained so far.

RETIN-A HINTS

You can dramatically improve the chance of Retin-A working for you by following a few simple guidelines:

—I recommend you apply Retin-A at night, before bed; then wash or shower it off in the morning.
—A few minutes before applying Retin-A, wash your face with a mild, nonastringent cleanser.
—Because Retin-A makes your skin effectively younger, and promotes the growth of new skin cells, your face also becomes that much more sensitive to sunlight. That means it is *essential* that you protect your new, tender (and youthful!) skin. *Always* wear an SPF (sun protection factor) 15 sunblock when you go out in the sun—even for a quick shopping trip. I tell my patients to get in the habit of putting on a sunblock each morning before they go out.
—It may also help to use a moisturizer each morning after you have removed the Retin-A. If you do, make sure it is a hypoallergenic product, to avoid irritating the tender new skin.

—If you are pregnant or nursing, do not use Retin-A.

—One consumers' advisory: Make sure you use the real thing. With the avalanche of press attention to tretinoin, several companies have jumped into the market to get their share of the pie, offering confusingly named products that are a far cry from what the doctor ordered. One such ersatz product calls itself Retinol-A, another Retinyl-A, and several others may have sprouted up by the time you read this. The truth is, there is no generic Retin-A, and the name of the only real product, made by Ortho Pharmaceutical Corporation, is Retin-A.

Retin-A has not yet been carefully tested in controlled experiments on large numbers of people, so we are still learning about its long-term effects. But it is already clear that Retin-A represents a quantum step in anti-aging skin care. It is an exciting step, and one which can make a difference in your own life and in the face that you see in the mirror! But keep three cardinal rules in mind:

—DON'T expect miraculous changes to happen overnight.

—DO expect an irritation reaction, particularly in the beginning.

—DO make Retin-A part of an overall skin-care team—not the only player.

What's Next?

Retin-A is only the first of what promises to be a new generation of skin-care creams. These products, the "cosmaceuticals," actually have proven medical effects and are more than simple moisturizers. Several other promising possibilities are now coming through the research pipeline, and will be appearing in the coming years.

Now that you have made Retin-A the first step of your young-skin program, let's look at what else you can do right now to keep your skin youthful.

Step Two: Moisturizers

When it comes to moisturizers, there is good news and bad news. First, the bad: None of the $10 billion worth of commercial cosmetics we buy each year really reverse the damages of age at the cellular level. Now the good news: They may make you look as if they do.

Moisturizers work on a simple principle. They keep water next to your skin, and as the moistened skin swells, it masks small wrinkles, blemishes, and imperfections. Wrinkles don't really go away, of course, because no real repair has been done. When you rinse off the cream, or the moisture evaporates, they are still there. Still, for simple cosmetic value, these products may deliver a lot of illusory bang for the buck. For that reason, there is no reason not to continue using them, if you like the way you look.

You should know, however, that none of the "high-priced spreads" containing exotic oils and ingredients necessarily do a much better job than such old-fashioned stand-bys as basic cold cream and petroleum jelly. Nivea and Vaseline are hardly romantic, but these heavy oils do as good a job as any to keep the skin moist.

Summary ▶ Moisturizers have a place in your young-skin regime, but none of them, neither the basics nor the most elegant and expensive concoctions, actually do anything to repair the underlying problem.

Step Three: C Is for Collagen

There is, however, one kind of cream that may be an exception to this rule because laboratory science suggests it gets to the root of the problem. A prime component of skin is the connective protein collagen. It now appears that vitamin C may actually strengthen and rejuvenate the collagen in your skin in several ways.

For ten years, laboratory researchers at Duke University have been working with vitamin C and skin cells. Their work suggests that in the test tube a topical application of vitamin C cream works to help skin synthesize vital new collagen, the essential component that is damaged by aging. While we do not yet have absolute proof that vitamin C works in the body, at least one cosmetic manufacturer, Avon, has created a vitamin C-based skin cream that delivers the ascorbic acid (vitamin C) where it does the most good: right on the aging skin cells. Similarly, vitamin C has been shown to inhibit certain skin cancers.

Summary ▶ Vitamin C cream can't hurt, and may be a valuable addition to your young-skin regimen.

Step Four: Youth-Preserving Skin Nutrition

In addition to vitamin C, there are two other vitamins that play an important role in making your skin young from the inside out. To understand why, it's necessary to understand the phenomenon called "cross-linking." When you are young and your skin is at its most supple, the strings of collagen protein it contains are relatively well formed and neat. But as you age, the accumulated damage of sun, chemicals, wind, smoke, and biological toxins tangle those protein strings. In cross-linking, the proteins can grab on to each other, linking molecules where they should not and generally getting very tangled. When that happens, your skin loses its elasticity and becomes rigid.

A good way to visualize cross-linking is imagine hanging twenty strips of sticky adhesive tape from your hand, and vigorously moving them around. As the tape strips touch, they stick and become tangled, until soon they bear very little resemblance to the twenty neat rows you started with. With this happening throughout your skin's connective tissue, no wonder it loses its youthful suppleness!

Scientists now believe that the antioxidant vitamins C, A, and E can help prevent and undo the cellular damage of cross-linking. They work, not just in your skin, but in all the body's tissues where cross-linking can occur: connective tissues, tendons, blood vessels, cornea, bones, and many organs. These vitamins can also help promote skin healing, reduce the formation of scar tissue, and give your skin and mucosal tissues the elements they need to grow healthily and smoothly.

THEY FORM THE CORE OF YOUR YOUTH PRESERVA-TION PROGRAM, and are essential for your skin's youthful appearance and long-term health. *Your vitamin-supplement program*

Youth Preservation Category	Vitamin C	Vitamin E	Beta-carotene*
A	2 grams	400 I.U.	12,000 I.U.
B	3 grams	400 I.U.	15,000 I.U.
C	4 grams	600 I.U.	17,500 I.U.
D	4 grams	600 I.U.	18,000 I.U.
E	5 grams	600 I.U.	20,000 I.U.

*An entirely safe form of vitamin A

is based on your score from the personal "Youth Quotient" Assessment quiz you took in Chapter 4. Turn to page 81, at the end of Chapter 4, to find your Youth Preservation Category. That category determines the level of nutritional help your skin needs.

Vitamin A vs. Beta-carotene

You may wonder if there is something missing from this picture. Why don't I prescribe vitamin A? After all, A is important for keeping your skin, eyes, and the mucosal linings of your body healthy. Even your nails, glands, hair, and teeth need enough A to stay healthy and attractive. Studies show that four out of ten Americans—especially blacks and Hispanics—do not consume the RDA (Recommended Daily Allowance) for vitamin A.

However, vitamin A can also be toxic. Because this fat-soluble vitamin is stored in your fat and liver, it can build up to dangerously high levels. Too much vitamin A can create severe complications, like gout, anemia, and worse. Happily, there is a safer way to make sure you get enough.

"Better Than A": Beta-carotene

The truth is, not all vitamin A is created equal. Ready-made vitamin A, called retinol, comes from animal sources. Another form, the carotenoids, is present also in plants. The most important of carotenoids is beta-carotene. This orange chemical is a first-stage form of vitamin A, called a "precursor." Your body converts beta-carotene into the vitamin A it needs. That means you can take beta-carotene into the vitamin A, enjoy its vital youth benefits, yet avoid the possible toxicity of regular vitamin A. (One study, at Harvard University, had 11,000 physicians taking as much as 30 milligrams of beta-carotene each day. I don't recommend such huge doses—but when it comes to safety, 11,000 Harvard doctors can't be too wrong!)

The point is, your body will convert just how much beta-carotene it needs into usable vitamin A, while naturally protecting you against a toxic overdose. This makes beta-carotene an "A-Plus" nutrient—all the benefits of vitamin A PLUS complete safety. That's why you should get used to taking the harmless, beta-carotene form of vitamin A.

Beta-carotene, like the other skin nutrients vitamins E and C, is a powerful antioxidant. It fights the free radicals that cause aging in your skin and throughout your body. At Harvard researchers have shown that beta-carotene may prevent or slow the development of skin cancer. Not only does beta-carotene fight biological damage to our cells as we age, it has even been shown to extend life expectancy in animals, from mice to men. That's why you must make sure to get enough of it.

You can boost your beta-carotene by eating foods like those shown below:

Beta-carotene–Rich Foods

Beets
Broccoli
Butternut squash
Carrots
Kale
Parsnips
Pumpkins
Spinach
Sweet potatoes
Tomatoes
Greens:
Chicory

Watercress
Dandelion
Mustard
Radish
Collard
Others:
Cantaloupe
Papaya
Vegetable soups
Milk
Fresh tomato sauce

If you follow the plan and eat at least one 3-ounce serving of green, red, or yellow vegetables a day, you'll be giving yourself enough beta-carotene to make your skin and your whole body look younger. Because beta-carotene helps protect against cancer and aging, it is one of the easiest and most delicious parts of your Youth Preservation prescription.

Summary ▶ Get sufficient vitamins C and E and beta-carotene from food and from the supplement regime I suggest, based on your Youth Preservation Category.

Step Five: The Sin of Sun

Mad dogs and Englishmen
go out in the midday sun.

—NOEL COWARD

This step has little to do with research breakthroughs or exotic treatments. It's news you've surely heard before. Yet it is *your single best and most effective way to keep your skin young.* The tip? Stay out of the sun. Period.

Sunlight—that seemingly promotes a "healthy" tan—works like a destructive time machine, giving you the skin of a person many decades older. When rays of light enter the skin cells, they react with oxygen, creating the free radicals we discussed earlier. These unstable oxygen molecules, in turn, damage virtually every aspect of your cells: membranes, fats, the proteins the cells need to operate, and the DNA and RNA they need to replicate. This process, called "photoaging," damages your skin in ways that normal aging does not:

—Changing its color from rosy red to yellowish
—Toughening, roughening, and wrinkling extensively
—Spotting with brown patches, red spidery veins, and warty growths
—Accelerates by many times the normal loss of elasticity

Of course, this is just the damage you can see. At the same time, overexposure to the sun increases your risk for three kinds of skin cancer, one of which, malignant melanoma, is especially deadly. If you think you've heard most of this before, stay tuned anyway because you probably haven't heard about two new wrinkles under the sun—more reasons that scientists have found that sunlight is bad news for those who want young skin.

Which is older?

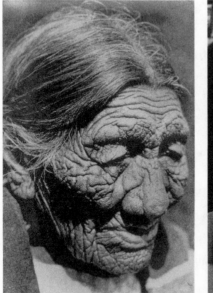 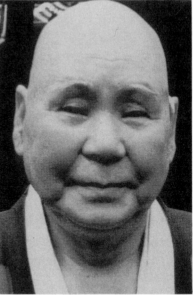

62-year-old American Indian woman   *91-year-old Tibetan monk*
with extensive sun exposure   *with very little sun exposure*

Courtesy Albert M. Kligman, M.D.

TRY THE "CHEEK-TO-CHEEK TEST"

Many of what we usually think of as the inevitable changes of aging are, in truth, the results of photoaging. You can see the dramatic proof of that through what I call the "cheek-to-cheek test." Compare the skin on your buttocks (that is, if you're not a habitual sunbather *au naturel*) with the skin on your face, arms, and hands. The skin that was covered shows what the "inevitable" and normal skin-aging process looks like. The difference between that and the more exposed skin areas is the price of indiscriminate photoaging—a price that is avoidable.

OZONE AND AGING

The ozone layer, ten to twenty miles above the planet's surface, may not seem very relevant to your life. But we now know it directly affects your chances of ending up with cancer and prematurely aged skin. The ozone layer works like a layer of sunscreen over the whole planet. This chemical blanket absorbs large amounts of ultraviolet radiation, preventing our sensitive skin from being bombarded by it.

Unfortunately, planet Earth's sunscreen is dissolving even as you read this. The protective ozone layer has decreased 3 percent in recent years, bringing a 15 percent rise in skin cancer cases. That means, 78,000 more people will get skin cancer, and more than 1,000 will die. It is because of the decrease in the ozone layer that the rate of skin cancer has never been higher. If the trend continues, as experts predict, we will see tens of thousands of new skin cancer cases, and thousands of needless, avoidable deaths.

Also, a Cornell Medical School study shows that too much sun can deplete your body's stores of the very beta-carotene that protects it. Another reason (if you needed one) to make sure you take adequate beta-carotene supplements.

Clearly, it is more important than ever to control the amount of sun your skin gets. However, that is probably not news to you. The real news is how to do it most effectively.

Summary ▶ Stay out of the sun as much as possible.

Step Six: Sunscreen, the Skin Savior

Most sunscreens do a good job of absorbing certain kinds of light rays—called "ultraviolet B (UVB)." That is the type of sunlight that gives you a burn. The UVB rays only penetrate your skin's top layers, and with most protective sunscreens, much of this radiation can be blocked. How much is blocked is what is meant by the sun protection factor (SPF) on the label of the bottle or tube.

But that's only half the story. Experts have recently come to understand that there is another villain responsible for sun aging, ultraviolet A (UVA) light. Where the UVB rays penetrate only the top layers of the skin, the more powerful UVA rays penetrate even deeper, damaging the deepest layers of the skin and the supporting collagen tissues.

Unfortunately, many of the commercial sunscreens use PABA

Skin Penetration of Light Rays

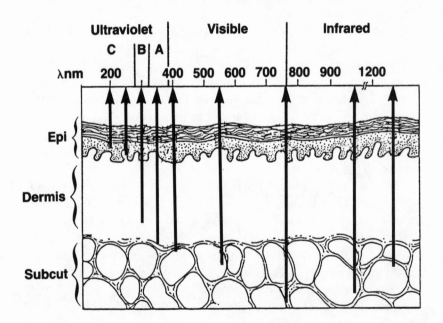

Paba vs. Natural Melanin Ultraviolet Protection

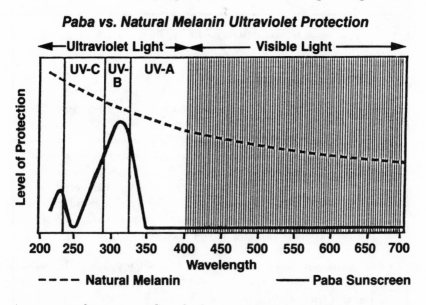

(para-aminobenzoic acid), which stops UVB but still lets most of the dangerous UVA penetrate to your skin's deepest levels. These creams prevent visible burning, so can lull you into a false sense of security: You stay out longer, exposed to harmful UVA rays. These rays not only increase the risk of skin cancer, but accelerate the aging of the deepest layers of the skin.

The only moderately effective sunscreens that work against UVA and UVB rays are those containing both PABA and a chemical called oxybenzone (by the time you read this, these preparations will be the majority on the market). Such "wide-spectrum" preparations represent the state-of-the-art in sun protection.

However, there is one thing you need to know about wide-spectrum creams. *The sun protection factor listed on the bottle or tube applies only to their UVB (sunburn) protection.* When it comes to the damaging UVA rays, their protection value is equivalent to about a 2. That means you have to use them with great care, for though they keep you from burning up to fifteen to thirty times longer, they only give you minimal protection against invisible aging damage, no matter what number is shown on the label. So, until more powerful wide-spectrum blockers are available, limiting sun exposure mechanically—with clothes, hats, and shade—is still the way to keep your skin supple, smooth, and young.

A NOTE ABOUT ALLERGIES . . .

You may have tried sunscreens with PABA or oxybenzone, found that you had a severe inflammation, or a burning or itching sensation when you went out into the sun, and concluded that you were allergic to PABA. You're probably half right—you may have an allergy but most likely, it's not to these ingredients. Laboratory tests show that fewer than one person in a thousand have documented allergic reactions to PABA.

But if you feel you are that one person, or you have especially sensitive skin that does have problems, you can shop around for products without PABA. It doesn't matter which other UVB sunscreen they contain: So long as you choose a suitable SPF, you'll be protected. I recommend that you try Sundown Broad Spectrum, because it uses titanium, which blocks UVA rays, and is free of PABA. However, if you have problems with one brand, always experiment with another until you find one you tolerate better.

Summary ▶ If you must be in the sun, use wide-spectrum sunscreens containing PABA and oxybenzone. If the PABA bothers your skin, switch to another sunscreen with an equal SPF number, and preferably one that contains oxybenzone for UVA protection.

Looking Ahead to Tomorrow's Breakthroughs . . .

Part of the task of this book is to alert you to research developments that, if they are not here yet, may be available soon. In the burgeoning field of anti-aging skin products, Retin-A represents only the first generation of true anti-aging treatments that actually reverse the process. The science of skin rejuvenation is exploding with even more exciting developments. As this book goes to press, a ferocious war is going on in research laboratories the world over to develop other, more powerful ways to rejuvenate the skin. Let me share with you some of the research breakthroughs that will change your life (or at least your skin's life) in the next few years. Remember—you heard it here first!

FACTOR X

From biomedical researchers in Denmark comes word of what may be the most promising new substance on the research horizon. Developed by the British biotechnology laboratory Senetek, it has a name that conjures images of secret laboratories and mysterious ingredients: Factor X. If early reports prove out, it may indeed be a stunning breakthrough in anti-aging treatment. Factor X may be nothing less than the biochemical fountain of youth that can prevent the changes that age causes in skin cell structure.

Normally, as the body's cells live longer, they change shape and their volume increases, so fewer of them can fit in the same space. The result is that the body's tissues become less compact—and biochemically less efficient. At the same time, older cells in the skin dramatically slow their production of critical cell proteins, such as elastin, that your skin needs to stay flexible, supple, and healthy.

Enter Factor X. When this extract is added to the cells and they are observed under a microscope, the changes that normally happen in older cells seem not to happen. They remain compact looking and, acting like younger cells, continue to churn out the critical proteins that help the skin stay young.

Clearly, such a product, if it proved viable, would represent a stunning breakthrough in the chemical treatment of aging—not just for the skin, but for cells throughout the body. Thus far, it is very hard to get much information about the project, and key details remain shrouded in secrecy. Dr. Nick Coppard, one of the biochemists in charge of the project, says only that they hope to begin human trials with an anti-aging skin lotion within the next year. They may have even begun by the time this book goes to press. Keep your eyes open for late-breaking news about how you can use Factor X to keep your skin looking younger, longer.

Looking ahead to future developments, there are several new products that could revolutionize how our skin ages.

Full-spectrum sunscreens that block the full range of skin-damaging ultraviolet light will be available. Versions of these that are already on the market are relatively crude; as we learn more about the UVA skin aging, we can expect to see safer and more effective sunscreens that will afford you high-range protection for the entire spectrum of ultraviolet radiation.

Genetically engineered sunscreen is being developed by a California laboratory called Advanced Polymer Systems. Utilizing a remarkable fusion of high-tech and natural approaches, this sunscreen contains the strongest natural sun protection known, the skin pigment melanin.

Melanin is the perfect sunscreen you would come up with if you were as smart as Mother Nature and had tens of millions of years to work in. This pigment shields you from wavelengths of ultraviolet light in direct proportion to their damaging effect on your skin. Studies show that black Africans, who have very high levels of natural melanin in their skin, have a "built-in" sun protection factor of 15. Soon, you may be able to benefit from the same protection.

Unfortunately, melanin has been too scarce to use—until now. California researchers have found a way to produce large quantities of natural, safe melanin using genetic engineering. However, melanin doesn't work effectively if you just slather it on, so other researchers have come up with an astonishing way to apply it where it does the most good.

They encapsulate it in tiny microscopic sponges, so infinitesimal that a single one measures about 1/1000th of an inch and weighs about 1/4 *billionth* of an ounce! These "microsponges" trap the genetically engineered melanin next to the skin, creating an effective, safe layer of the natural pigment that Nature meant you to have.

This radical approach promises a safer, more effective, natural sunscreen. Though the project is still on the drawing board, look for the first melanin products in the early 1990s.

Sun protection in a pill. What would have sounded like science fiction just a few years ago is being investigated and developed in research centers around the country. The goal: sunscreen products you swallow instead of applying.

Researchers at the University of Arizona Medical Center are working on a way to boost your body's own sun-protection mechanism: a tanning hormone that increases the natural melanin. They have created a superactive analog of a natural hormone called "melanocyte stimulating hormone" (MSH), which "instructs" the body to manufacture more pigment cells in the skin. Biochemi-

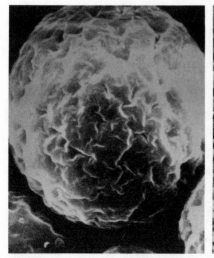 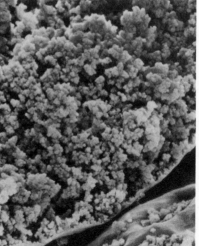

Melanin-containing Microsponges™ magnified 5,000 times (actual diameter: 1/1000 of an inch)

Cross-section interior of Microsponges™. One gram of these sponges contains 240,000 miles of melanin-containing tunnels.

Advanced Polymer Systems

cally, it is the same reaction that occurs when a chameleon changes color—or when you get a natural tan. This hormone would make your skin look as if you had been at the beach all summer—but with none of the serious aging effects that would create. The goal is not just to make you look naturally healthy and fit (though you would), but to block sunlight so it doesn't penetrate to damage and age the deeper skin tissues. Early tests suggest that the hormone product is nontoxic and could be swallowed like a pill.

The protective tan MSH creates may last as long as several months—guarding you against the sun, reducing your risk of skin cancer, and giving you a glowing, appealing tan. The research is only in its earliest phase in animals, so don't expect to see these products on the market for at least six or seven years. But if MSH works, it will be among the hottest news on the scientific horizon.

Scientists at Harvard Medical School are trying a very different approach. Instead of blocking the sun from striking the skin cells, as with lotions, or filtering it with the skin's own pigment, they are trying to help the body repair the damage that light can cause within the skin itself. A photobiologist in Boston reports early laboratory research based on the theory of anti-oxidants, which are thought to be key to many of the body's aging processes. The goal is to neutralize the deadly oxygen by-products—the free radicals—which are created in your cells by exposure to ultraviolet light. Because free radicals cause skin aging, cross-linking, and skin cancer, researchers hope that by chemically inactivating these destructive oxygen molecules, tissue damage can be prevented before it happens. They envision using this kind of pill not as a replacement for the bottle of sunscreen at the beach, but as protection against limited short-duration exposures to sun.

"Sun protection in a pill" is one of the most exciting and creative ideas on the anti-aging horizon. Laboratories are trying to perfect the first generation of oral sun protectors. The medical evidence all points to one inescapable conclusion: *Within the next few years, we will have a stunning new array of tools that not only control, but reverse disfiguring skin aging.*

The Six-Step Skin-Care Program

However, in order to take full advantage of these new developments, you must do all you can now to keep your skin young, using every tool at your disposal today. Your prescription is to heed the six vital steps to skin rejuvenation . . . starting right now! Include these six crucial steps in your younger-skin regimen:

1. Ask your doctor if you are a candidate for Retin-A cream.
2. If you use a basic moisturizer, do it only for cosmetic, not therapeutic, results.
3. Consider using a nutrient-enriched (vitamin C) skin cream.
4. Take an appropriate Youth Preservation nutrient regime (as determined by your personal Youth Preservation Quotient), and keep your diet high in beta-carotene.
5. Keep out of the sun as much as possible. Period.
6. If you use a sunblock, use one that contains a wide-spectrum PABA-oxybenzone agent.

6
Young at Heart: Building Yourself a State-of-the-Art Heart

Heart disease before eighty is our own fault, not God's or Nature's will.
—HARVARD UNIVERSITY CARDIAC SPECIALIST
PAUL DUDLEY WHITE, M.D.

ENERGY. FITNESS. VIGOR. They are synonymous with all it means to be youthful. For true biological youth has little to do with how many birthdays you have chalked up. What counts is your vitality, how you can bound up a flight of stairs or enjoy playing with a child or grandchild with energy and full enjoyment. It means waking to each day brimming with vigor and enthusiasm, knowing you can count on your body to perform what you demand of it, knowing it will deliver the energy, vitality, and stamina you need to lead an active life.

All of that depends on one muscle—the one beating in your chest right now. You are only as youthful as your heart is, and this essential muscle determines your vitality, how young you feel, and whether you will have the breath, energy, and stamina to meet life on your terms. It is an essential component not just of longevity, but of a truly healthy, vital existence.

A too-old heart makes you too old to enjoy the wonderful bounty that life holds for those who have the vitality to seize it. Premature heart aging robs more than five million Americans of this vitality, makes them sluggish and sedentary, and steals years from their productive, active lives. They weaken or die too young with a heart that is too old; the victims of 100 percent preventable, 100 percent unnecessary cardiovascular aging.

But this unnecessary killer disease doesn't happen so much to people in other societies, and it won't happen to you if you follow the guidelines I recommend. Below are the six easy steps you need to keep your heart strong and sound, pumping forcefully and faithfully, assuring you of decades of active, positive life. They are the state-of-the-medical art in preventive cardiology, geared to add several years to the life of your heart. Follow them and I promise you: One year from today, your heart will be "younger" than it is today. You will have a 100 percent state-of-the-art heart!

1. STOP SMOKING NOW, TO REJUVENATE YOUR HEART.
2. EAT A "HEART-SMART" DIET THAT REDUCES SATU-RATED FATS.
3. CONSUME FISH AS A MAIN MEAL AT LEAST TWICE WEEKLY. AVOID FRIED FISH.
4. EAT FIBER TO REDUCE FATS AND CHOLESTEROL.
5. TAKE TIME EACH DAY TO RELAX AND REDUCE STRESS.
6. GET MODERATE EXERCISE AND ACTIVITY SEVERAL TIMES A WEEK.

With these steps you can do *more* than just prevent your heart from aging. You can actually *reverse* destructive heart and artery changes that may have already occurred.

Much of this may sound familiar. That's fine. Our goal is to help you incorporate these cardio-fitness rules into a life-prolonging, health-prolonging plan—to make you 100 percent "young at heart."

A Heart Choice

It has been said that the average American's heart loses up to one third of its pumping capacity by age seventy. *But new research shows that such a cardiac decline is neither inevitable nor necessarily built in.* Maintain your heart right, and it will work

Two Views of Heart Longevity

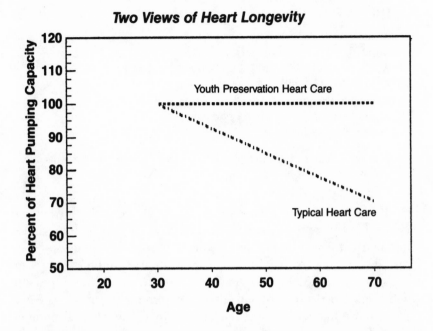

about as well at age eighty as it did at twenty. Heart decay occurs, not because of normal aging, but because of a lifetime of cardiac ignorance, mistreatment, or abuse. It's up to you: Which lifeline do *you* want to be on?

Summary ▶ The loss of heart function with age is not "natural." It *is* preventable. Staying young at heart is up to you.

Test Yourself: How Old Is Your Heart?

The greater your present risk for cardiac disease, the older the effective age of your heart and cardiovascular system. Are you:

GROUP A:

From a family with a history of heart disease?   ——
A smoker?   ——
With cholesterol above 230?   ——
With blood pressure above 140/90? (If so, see special note on page 117.)   ——

GROUP B:

A diabetic? _____
More than 15% overweight? _____
A survivor of one or more heart attacks? _____
Ever diagnosed with angina? _____
Suffering occasional sharp chest pains? _____
A competitive, hard-driving personality? _____
Sedentary and inactive? _____

For each Yes answer in Group A, add two years to your cardiac age.
For each Yes answer in Group B, add one year to your cardiac age.

If you have any of the factors in Group A, your risk for having heart disease, and perhaps a heart attack, is two to four times higher than if you don't. The factors in Group B are less severe, but also increase your risk for heart disease. Combine factors in both groups, and the risk increases that much more. A person with high blood pressure and high cholesterol who smokes is *eight times* more likely to have a heart attack than one who has none of these factors.

The good news is that *you can change most of these factors.*

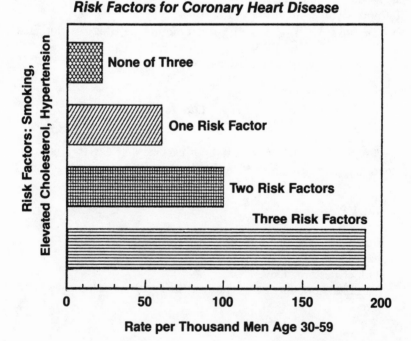

Risk Factors for Coronary Heart Disease

You have the chance to reap the wonderful rewards of being youthful, energetic, and strong at heart for many years to come!

Young-at-Heart Step One:
Where There's Smoke, There's Danger

Do you know the *single most effective* way to reduce your heart's age? Stop smoking. Right now. There is no better way to dramatically and significantly lower the effective age of your entire cardiovascular system. Consider:

—The heart disease rate is twice as high in smokers than in nonsmokers—four times as high for heavy smokers.
—Smokers are at higher risk for sudden death, heart attack, artery disease, and aneurysm, and are twice as likely to have a stroke as nonsmokers.
—Smoking ages virtually every part of the cardiovascular system prematurely and unnecessarily.

Happily, just as soon as you stop smoking, your risk begins dropping sharply, so that after five years, you are at no higher

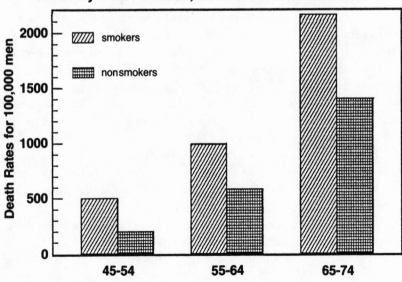

Coronary Heart Disease, Smokers vs. Nonsmokers

risk for stroke than a nonsmoker. After ten years, if you smoked less than a pack a day, your heart risk would be virtually identical to that of someone who never smoked. *Every day you don't smoke, your heart heals itself and gets younger!* Stopping smoking *now* is the single most dramatic step you can take to make your cardiovascular system effectively younger. Period.

Summary ▶ The sooner you stop smoking, the sooner your body will rebuild your heart.

Young-at-Heart Step Two:
Clean out Those Pipes

Diet can influence your long-term health prospects more than any other action. Of greatest concern is our intake of dietary fat for chronic diseases such as coronary artery disease . . . and strokes.—U.S. Surgeon General's Report on Nutrition and Health, 1988

The Surgeon General, our highest health authority, has finally said what many have known for some time: Diet is the most important tool against heart aging. National health authorities have now made "less fat" America's number-one diet priority.

Yet the National Institutes of Health reports that most Americans' cholesterol levels are still too high. That means that, although the basic goal is clear, people are confused about how to put dietary recommendations into practice. They hear "high-density lipoproteins" and "low-density lipoproteins"; "triglycerides" versus "cholesterol"; "saturated," "polyunsaturated," and "monosaturated" fats—and end up befuddled about what they ought to eat, *right now*, to make a difference.

Enough. If you want to keep your cardiovascular system young, if you want to enjoy the health and longevity advantages of a state-of-the-art heart, remember this one simple principle: *Keep your pipes clear and clean.*

A young circulatory system is one whose arterial pipelines are smooth and unblocked, with the least possible arterial thickening and blood-blocking plaque deposits. The cleaner, more fat-free you keep your blood, the more you reverse aging in arteries, veins, and heart. Every percent you lower your blood cholesterol means

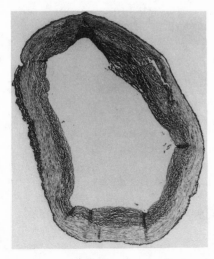

Normal coronary artery cross-section

*Coronary artery clogged with
fatty buildup*

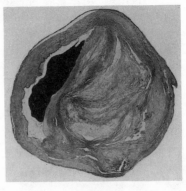

Courtesy of American Heart Association

a 2 percent drop in your heart-attack risk. What could be simpler?

On page 112 are nine basic diet principles, based on recommendations of the National Institutes of Health, the American Heart Association, and virtually every responsible cardio-health authority. Follow these rules, and every bite you take will help you strip away years from the biological age of your cardiovascular system.

This plan has helped thousands of my patients give themselves a cardiac "retread." It has given them state-of-the-art hearts to make them feel more buoyant and energetic, more alive and vigorous. They feel more alive, can exercise (some for the first time in years!) and have more energy for work, hobbies, and family. With these nine diet rules you can turn back the clock on aging, remove previously deposited fats from your artery walls, give your cardiovascular system a "retread"—and ensure a longer, more vigorous life. You can see why I want *you* to start experiencing such terrific benefits!

Nine Diet Rules for a
State-of-the-Art Heart

1. Increase your intake of complex carbohydrates (starches).
2. Greatly reduce red meats and animal fats and trim off all visible fat.
3. Eat fewer eggs or eggs without the yolks.
4. Eat more fish. Try for three times each week.
5. When you do eat fats, make sure they are monosaturated, not saturated or polyunsaturated (see Appendix A, "Cardiac Longevity Foods").
6. Increase your fiber intake—whole grains, fresh fruits, and vegetables. You should eat fiber with every meal.
7. Reduce consumption of highly refined foods, including refined sugar.
8. Instead of fried foods, eat broiled, baked or boiled foods.
9. Reduce your intake of coffee.

Summary ▶ Reduce saturated fats and cholesterol in your diet.

Turning Back the Clock

By themselves, these tips aren't radical. What is radical is how they can actually reverse heart and arterial damage that may have already occurred, and effectively drop your cardiac age.

Let me explain. Cholesterol circulates in your body by piggybacking on one of two one-way messengers: LDL (low-density lipoprotein) moves cholesterol from your liver to your tissues and organs (like your cardiac vessels); HDL (high-density lipoprotein) transports it back. By changing the ratio of those elements, with more HDL carrying cholesterol back to the liver and less LDL carrying it out to the blood vessels, you can halt the process that ages the heart and arteries. The single best way to do that is through the ratio of saturated fat and cholesterol you eat.

Research shows that if you lower your LDL level to below 100, your body can actually start pulling deposited fats and cholesterol out of your blood vessel walls, so they can heal them-

Cholesterol Transport in the Body

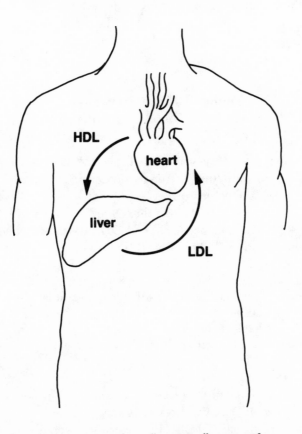

selves and return to a smoother, "younger" state. That means heart rejuvenation, pure and simple, allowing your heart and arteries to function as long and well as Nature designed them to.

By lowering your total cholesterol and reducing your LDL, *you can actually reverse the damage accumulated before you ever picked up this book!* In six months your blood vessels will actually look smoother, more open and elastic—*younger* in every biochemical sense—than they are right now.

New Surprise: Coffee and Cholesterol?

Brand-new research in the *American Journal of Epidemiology* suggests that coffee drinking may raise your cholesterol. Interestingly, no such link has been found for tea, colas, or other caffeine-containing drinks, or even for decaffeinated coffee. However, something in coffee seems to cause this problem. Until we know just what it is, it appears that drinking less java means a younger heart.

Young-at-Heart Step Three: Make Your Diet More E-Fish-Ent

Next comes an easy way to balance the fats in your blood. *Starting today, with this evening's dinner, eat fish at least two times each week.* Doctor's orders.

Fish contains the best fats, the Omega-3 fatty acids, among them EPA (eicosapentaenoic acid) and DHA (docosahexaenoic acid). Among their many positive effects, they:

—Make your blood platelets less sticky
—Reduce several chemical steps that lead to arterial lesions
—Reduce LDL levels
—Reduce overall cholesterol
—Reduce blood pressure
—Minimize inflammation

They are your key to achieving a clean, smooth, youthful heart and blood system. You will greatly reduce your risk of early death from coronary disease. Fish oils have also been shown to help people who have had their arteries opened surgically to keep them clear, and young. Obviously, you should have your fish dishes broiled, baked, poached, or boiled—not fried.

Fish oil works best when it is eaten as fish rather than as pills. There is less risk of side effects or overdosing; you have one less pill to take, and using fish as your protein source means you will be eating less meat, whose saturated fats boost cholesterol. And fish is so much more delicious!

Summary ▶ Eat fish as a main meal at least twice weekly. Avoid fried fish.

Young-at-Heart Step Four:
Fiber for Your Heart

You may think fiber helps with bowel regularity, or weight loss, or even as cancer protection—and it does. But it also reduces excess blood fats and cholesterol.

Fiber helps prevent your body from absorbing the wrong fats from foods. Its chemical and mechanical action sweeps unhealthy fats out of your intestines, reducing cholesterol that would otherwise gum up your blood, blood vessels, and heart.

People in societies that consume high levels of fiber have significantly younger hearts and low rates of cardiovascular aging. The Japanese, who eat more fiber per capita than any other nation, lose one seventh as many people to heart attacks as we do in the United States, which has one of the world's lowest rates of fiber consumption. In America vegetarians who eat a lot of fiber have less fat in their blood, and lower average blood pressures, than people with low-fiber intake. A high-fiber diet can lower triglycerides and cholesterol by one fifth to one third, slowing down the aging of your entire cardiac system.

When it comes to clearing out fat, not all fiber is created equal. I especially recommend:

—Soybean fiber, which has been shown to significantly decrease cholesterol in people with moderately high levels.

—Oat bran, which is also highly effective. Get in the habit of starting your day with a bowl of regular (not instant) oatmeal.

—Corn fiber, which is one of the newest food supplements, and has been shown to reduce cholesterol by an average of 20 percent, and other blood fats by more than 30 percent. Even better, this insoluble fiber has very few calories.

—Guar gum is another terrific blood fat-fighter. A Stanford University study shows that guar-gum supplements reduce both the overall cholesterol level and the specific type of cholesterol (LDL) most implicated in aging your heart and blood vessels. I have given many of my patients these supplements to reduce high cholesterol, blood fats, and with them, the age of their cardiovascular system.

—A natural fiber preparation called "psyllium hydrophilic mucil-loid," available at your local pharmacy, is also effective in lowering cholesterol.

Other fiber sources that can extend the life of your heart are:

Fiber Sources to Fight Cardio-aging		
Fiber class	Found in these foods	Absorbs fats & cholesterol
Pectin	Apples, grapes, potatoes, squash, oranges, lemons, grapefruit	Yes
Gum	Oats, oat bran, barley, lentils, chick-peas, black-eyed peas, pinto beans, navy beans, split peas	Yes
Mucilage	Seeds	Yes

In addition, many fiber foods are good sources of vitamins, such as vitamin C and the B vitamin inositol, which your body needs to fight fats and cholesterol.

Diet Before Drugs

Eating the proper food is always your first and best line of defense against early heart aging. Only if you cannot achieve results with diet alone should your doctor prescribe drugs to help lower your cholesterol. Some of these drugs (called "bile-seques-trants," such as cholestyramine or colestipol) prevent the cholesterol from being absorbed from your digestive tract in the first place, and some of them (such as lovastatin) work in the blood-stream itself.

You should ask your doctor for the first kind. According to the National Heart, Lung, and Blood Institute, bile-sequestrant drugs should be the first treatment after diet; they are preferable to drugs that work in the bloodstream. If you must use medication, discuss the different options with your doctor.

But remember: By following the guidelines in this chapter, you should need no drugs at all. To get you started, I have included a special appendix section at the end of this book, with a specific state-of-the-art heart diet, and extensive information on heart-preservative fiber-rich foods.

Summary ▶ Use fiber and diet—not drugs—to reduce fats and cholesterol.

SPECIAL NOTE FOR HYPERTENSIVES . . .

We can't talk about keeping your heart young without a word about blood pressure. If you answered yes to the question about blood pressure in the self-test on page 107, you may be the one in six Americans who has hypertension. That puts you at higher risk for several diseases, including heart attack and stroke. In addition, your cardiovascular system is aging faster than it should.

BLOOD PRESSURE MYTH

Many people seem to think you can tell persons with high blood pressure because they are nervous, jittery, or tense. That is more myth than medicine. Hypertension and personality bear no relation to each other. People with high blood pressure can be tense and anxious or placid and laid-back.

Usually you can do something about high blood pressure. With your doctor's help, you can probably remove yourself from this risk group completely. But to start, here are three heart-helping hints to lower your blood pressure, your risk for stroke and heart attack—and your biological age.

First—Reduce the alcohol you drink. If it's two drinks a day, make it one. Try some nonalcoholic beverages, or dilute the alcohol you do drink with mixers. This is an absolutely necessary step to reducing the excess blood pressure that is prematurely aging your circulatory system.

Second—Stop using salt on your food, and start paying careful attention to the salt content of the prepared, frozen, and canned foods you eat. Make sodium-free salt substitutes a part of your diet. Expand your taste in seasoning to include garlic, onions, and herbs in place of salt in every dish. You've probably heard those two tips before (from your own physician, I hope!), but you may not have heard this final recommendation.

Third—Eat more fiber, the natural way to control blood pressure. It has been shown that when low-fiber eaters include more of it in their diet for one month, their blood pressure drops significantly. Many natural forms of fiber—vegetables and grains— also include minerals like magnesium, calcium, and potassium, which also help stabilize blood pressure.

All three of these heart-helping hints are essential to controlling this insidious and common factor responsible for aging your body before its time. After following these tips for a month, check yourself against this chart:

Age	Average Male Blood Pressure	Average Female Blood Pressure
25	124/76 E	
30	125/76 E	
35	125/80 E	115/75 F
40	128/82 F 129/81 E	119/75 F
45	130/83 F	125/78 F
50	134/83	130/81 F
55	134/83 F	139/83 F
60	136/82 F 140/83 E	148/84 F

If your blood pressure is still too high, talk with your doctor to see if you are a candidate for blood-pressure-lowering medicine. Remember: You *can* eliminate high blood pressure, and by removing this premature aging factor from your life, you take a large step toward extending your most healthy and vigorous years.

Young-at-Heart Step Five:
A Calm Heart Is a Young Heart

The next step is both simple and very difficult. Relax. We have long known that too much stress puts you at risk for heart attack. Who can't recall being under stress and feeling their heart thumping or racing? Unfortunately, that is just the visible sign of the serious long-term effects stress puts on your heart:

—Men with what doctors term the "Type A" personality—hard-driving, impatient, achieving, competitive—are twice as likely to develop heart disease as their calmer, "Type B" fellows.

—Those who have lost a spouse to death are much more at risk for heart attack than are their same-age friends who have not experienced emotional trauma.

—Residents near major airports, living with the steady stress of aircraft noise, have high rates of heart disease and hypertension.

—From the *New England Journal of Medicine*, research shows that everyday stresses—acts as simple as talking about an emotional subject, doing math problems, or speaking in public—could trigger episodes of oxygen deprivation and erratic heartbeat. Though silent and painless, these episodes are nonetheless damaging.

—As this chapter went to press, a report in the *American Heart Journal* showed that psychological stress can lead to heart-rhythm abnormalities, and even fatal heart malfunction.

The evidence is clear: Stress weakens your heart, aging it before its time. Heart youth means reducing stress, to rejuvenate your heart.

WHAT'S YOUR "STRESS LOAD"?

Stress is very individual. What may seem a killing amount for one person might seem just about average for a second, and not bother a third person at all. We even require a certain amount of stress in our lives to feel motivated and stimulated. It is not the absolute level of stress that counts, but how you experience it—

your "stress load." This following quiz was designed for the U.S. Department of Health and Human Services to help you assess your stress load:

1. Do you have a supportive family? Yes ____ (10) No ____ (0)
2. Do you belong to a nonfamily social activity group, meeting at least once each month? Yes ____ (10) No ____ (0)
3. In a week, do you do something you really enjoy that is just for you? Yes ____ (5) No ____ (0)
4. At home, do you have a place to relax or be by yourself? Yes ____ (10) No ____ (0)
5. How often do you bring work home at night? ____ (multiply by −5)
6. Do you actively pursue a hobby? Yes ____ (10) No ____ (0)
7. Do you engage in deep relaxation (meditation, yoga, etc.) at least three times each week? Yes ____ (15) No ____ (0)
8. How many packs of cigarettes do you smoke each day? (multiply by 10)

   None ____
   One· ____
   Two ____
   Three or more ____

9. How many evenings each week do you use a drug or a drink to help fall asleep? ____ (multiply by −5)
10. Do you use a drug or drinks to help calm down during the day? ____ (multiply by −10)
11. How many times do you exercise 30 minutes or longer in a given week?

    I don't ____ (0)
    One ____ (5)
    Two ____ (10)
    Three ____ (15)
    Four or more ____ (20)

12. How many nutritionally balanced and wholesome meals do you eat each day?

    None ____ (0)
    One ____ (5)
    Two ____ (10)
    Three ____ (15)

13. Are you within five pounds of your "ideal" body weight for your age and bone type? Yes ____ (15) No ____ (0)
14. Do you practice time management techniques in your daily life? Yes ____ (10) No ____ (0)

    TOTAL SCORE: _____

SCORING:

100–120 Congratulations! You take care of your stress load well enough that you are not a candidate for stress-related heart aging.

60–100 You deal with stress adequately, but you have room to improve. Your heart could be having stress damage.

Below 60 Your stress levels are unhealthy. You risk aging your heart prematurely.

Now, let's improve things. Go back and look at the test questions. Each suggests a way you can build stress out of your life and give yourself a younger heart! You might:

1. Take up a hobby you enjoy.
2. Join a group that lets you get out with friends regularly.
3. Work to bring yourself within five pounds of your "ideal" weight.
4. Do some form of deep relaxation (meditation, yoga, biofeedback, etc.)
5. Make sure you get exercise every few days.
6. Learn to eat nutritionally balanced and wholesome meals.
7. Take time each week to do something special just for yourself.
8. Create a place to relax or be by yourself at home or nearby.
9. Learn and use time management techniques in your daily life.
10. Stop smoking (but you knew that!).
11. Learn to use relaxation exercises instead of alcohol or drugs to unwind before sleep.
12. Don't bring work home at night.

Do such measures work? Yes, says an intriguing study released from the Medical School of Athens. Epidemiologists, ruling out other known risk factors, found that men who took a half-hour nap daily to control stress were 30 percent less likely to suffer from coronary disease than men who didn't! Studies at Harvard show that relaxation exercises can help regulate irregular heartbeats in people with heart damage. Obviously, you don't have to take a siesta each day religiously, but some form of stress control will help take years off your heart.

Summary ▶ Taking time each day to relax and reduce stress keeps your heart young.

Young-at-Heart Step Six: Exercise

This last is a very simple, and very essential, point. *Every hour that you sit or lie around instead of being active shortens your life.* Period. While almost every part of your body benefits from exercise, by far the most good comes in your heart and circulatory system. Exercise can:

—Reduce bad LDL fats and increase good HDL fats.
—Reduce blood pressure in sedentary people.
—Help vanquish angina (heart pain due to lack of oxygen).
—Lower the risk of heart attack by more than half.
—Decrease excess body fat, which otherwise weakens your heart and shortens your life.
—Help you live longer.

Workers in high-activity jobs have less coronary artery disease than their low-activity colleagues. In the words of one textbook: "When people remain active, their body . . . tends to resemble that of younger people." The research message is clear—need I say more?

Well, yes. There are two myths about exercise that may be preventing you from taking advantage of its full heart-rejuvenating potential. Let's put them to rest.

EXERCISE MYTH #1: "You have to do serious aerobic workouts, marathons, and the like to benefit. I'm no athlete."

You don't have to be. The fact is, any exercise is better than none. Among the kinds of exercise that have been shown effective are:

Playing with children
Walking to errands
Cleaning windows
Vacuuming or mopping the floor
Bowling
Golf
Cleaning out the attic or cellar

Pruning trees
Body surfing
Gardening
Raking leaves
Dancing
Taking a hike
Playing
Climbing stairs
Mowing the lawn
Walking the dog
Swimming

This list proves the point: Any time spent being active is better than time spent not being active. If you expend even 1,000 calories each week above your daily needs, you begin to derive clear health benefits. You don't have to be a Greg Louganis or Carl Lewis, you just have to *not* be a couch potato. To be sure, if you are a more avid athlete, your potential benefit is that much greater. But just because you can't run a marathon is no reason to give up on the solid benefits of moderate activity to keep your heart young.

EXERCISE MYTH #2: "I'm too old to exercise. I can't make up for a life of not exercising."

Banish another myth. In truth, a reasonable program of activity and exercise will make you younger at any age. Researchers from the Palo Alto (California) Clinic measured age against one common laboratory standard of aging, the maximum oxygen uptake (VO_2Max), and found:

> If an inactive 70-year old were to begin an exercise program of "moderate activity," the result would be a gain of 15 years. . . . If the subject were to achieve the "athlete" level of conditioning, there would be a potential improvement of *40 years* [emphasis in original].—*Journal of American Geriatrics*

If that can work for seventy-year olds, think what it can do for you! As I sat down to write this chapter, a study was just published from the famed Honolulu Heart Program at Kauakini Medical

Center. They found that even among people forty-five to sixty-four years old, those who led active lives had almost one third less coronary heart disease than their inactive counterparts. Those men have functionally younger hearts, and can expect to live longer and better. Tennis, anyone?

Summary ▶ Moderate exercise and activity are crucial to giving yourself a state-of-the-art heart.

Looking Ahead: Tomorrow's State-of-the-Art Heart

—One of the most innovative and exciting weapons in our fight against high cholesterol came recently when the FDA approved a new "cholesterol card" test. You simply prick your finger and squeeze a drop of blood on the card, which changes color to signal if your cholesterol levels are in the low/safe, medium/normal, or high/danger range. As of this writing, the card is available only to doctors. But there are plans to license it for home use as well, and I hope it will be available by the time you read this. It is a quick, almost painless, and inexpensive means of assessing your own cholesterol risk.

—From Boston University and Harvard medical schools, a new discovery uses the natural vegetable compound beta-carotene to boost the most advanced laser-surgery techniques for clogged arteries. Powerful laser scalpels have proven difficult to use to open clogged arteries because they can also damage the surrounding blood vessel walls. But by treating patients with beta-carotene before surgery, doctors can alter the fatty deposits in the heart arteries, making them more vulnerable to laser light. Combining this natural vitamin and high-tech lasers, surgeons can vaporize dangerous fat deposits more easily without harming adjacent blood vessel walls.

—Some 500,000 Americans have an inherited defect in their cholesterol regulation system that predisposes them to heart attack. At the University of California at San Diego, researchers are working on a gene transplant that would replace those defective genes with biologically correct ones. If the experiment works, they will be able to inject these "corrected" genes, to be incorporated into a person's own genetic code. The hope is that as these new genes grow to replace an individual's own faulty genes, they will help clear excess cholesterol from the body.

—Scientists at Johns Hopkins University are working to develop a new breed of diagnostic tool, a miniaturized electronic capsule

that can be swallowed. Like a tiny internal satellite, once inside the body it sends radio signals that trace the heartbeat from the inside out. Such capsules may just be a first step: One day, electronics that you swallow may give you and your physician a more accurate, in-depth look at cardiac functioning than is now possible. The earliest prototypes may undergo testing in three years.
—Promising new drug research may hold good news for the sixty million Americans with high blood pressure. Radically different kinds of drugs, called "renin blockers," are now being perfected in Upjohn's research laboratories. They work on a new principle: They bind a million times more strongly to blood pressure enzymes than the body's own natural chemicals do, so they interfere with the runaway hypertension syndrome—before it turns dangerous. This drug may be generally available approximately five years from now.

Young-at-Heart Review

Remember the basic building blocks of a state-of-the-art heart:

1. THE LOSS OF HEART FUNCTION WITH AGE IS NOT "NATURAL." IT *IS* LARGELY PREVENTABLE.
2. STOP SMOKING NOW, TO REJUVENATE YOUR HEART.
3. REDUCE SATURATED FATS IN YOUR DIET.
4. EAT FISH AS A MAIN MEAL AT LEAST TWICE WEEKLY. AVOID FRIED FISH.
5. USE FIBER TO REDUCE FATS AND CHOLESTEROL.
6. TAKE TIME EACH DAY TO RELAX AND REDUCE STRESS.
7. GET MODERATE EXERCISE AND ACTIVITY SEVERAL TIMES A WEEK.

7

Where There's Smoke . . . There's Aging

Cigarettes are the most important individual health risk in this country, responsible for more premature deaths and disability than any other known agent.

—C. EVERETT KOOP, M.D.
U.S. SURGEON GENERAL

WELCOME TO THE briefest chapter of this book. If you are one of the fifty-four million Americans who still smoke, I wrote it just for you. If you're not, you can read it if you wish or skip ahead to the next chapter.

You may not be surprised that the message of this short chapter can be reduced to two short words: Stop Now. Simply put, smoking is one of the most effective ways to age your body prematurely and cause you to die too young. *This means that to stop smoking is one of the most effective steps you can take to slow the aging process throughout your body.*

Smoking works against every single principle of this book, and defeats your goal of living longer and more healthily. If you have a two-pack-a-day habit, you have a 70 percent greater chance of dying of disease than your friends who don't smoke, and you can expect to shorten your life by eight to nine years. In this case, the charts on the next page are worth a thousand words:

I expect you already know all of this. But what you may not know is that there is a real silver lining for you behind these grim

127

Longevity of Male Smokers and Nonsmokers, from Age 35

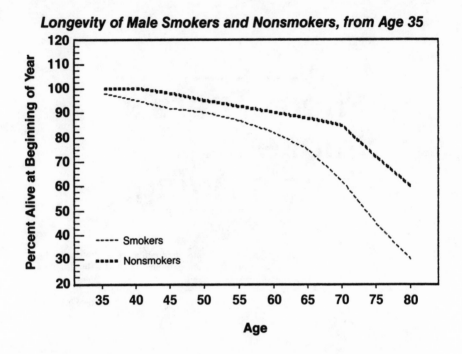

Longer Life for Former Smokers, Male and Female

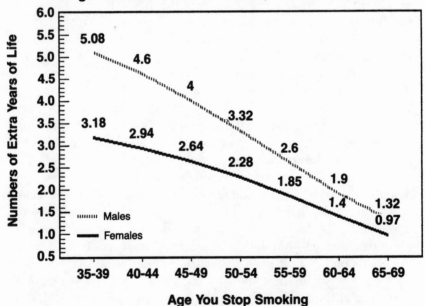

statistics. *As a smoker, you are in a unique position to make an immense positive change in your life expectancy.* If this book motivates you to do nothing but stop smoking, that one change means a 100 percent guaranteed, 100 percent positive impact on your longevity. By that single act, you will have won yourself more years of life and better years of health than through any other life change you can make.

Age That You Stop Smoking

Of course, it isn't just how long you live, but how well. By stopping smoking now you will have more stamina and endurance, clearer breathing, fewer infections and colds, younger-looking skin, and significantly better physical energy and vitality.

Summary ▶ Stopping smoking guarantees better health and longevity.

I don't want to dwell on what you've already heard about the dangers of smoking. Instead, I want to give you some information that you may not have heard—and a specific four-part program to help you stop.

Part One: Just the Facts

Research shows that accurate information is a big part of helping you stop smoking. So, your first step to enjoying a healthy, long, smoke-free life is to get the most well-rounded picture of what smoking does to your health. *This information is the first step in your commitment to stopping smoking.*

You know that quitting now will give you a younger heart and cardiovascular system. You probably know, too, that the same is true of your lungs. Because smoking increases your risk for lung cancer between ten and twenty-five times, stopping now removes you from these risk groups—increasing your longevity potential still further.

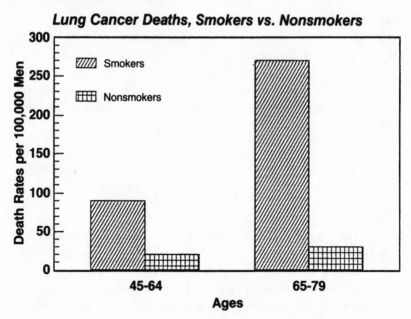

Lung Cancer Deaths, Smokers vs. Nonsmokers

While stopping smoking rejuvenates your heart and lungs, and increases your life span, it also decreases the risks shown opposite.

What better way to rejuvenate and protect so many areas of the body—Just Say No to Tobacco!

FOR MOTHERS ONLY

For pregnant women, smoking has special risks (page 132).

Add these factors up, then figure in the severe aging effects smoking has on your heart and blood vessels, and you begin to see why it is the single most pernicious cause of early mortality we know, one that takes 315,000 lives every year. But more important, it points the way to *the obvious step you can take right now* to easily, simply, give yourself years of extra-quality life. Knowing the whole health story, you know that *you can choose to build these problems out of your life.* So what are you waiting for?

Summary ▶ Knowing all the facts is the first part to quitting.

Effects of Smoking

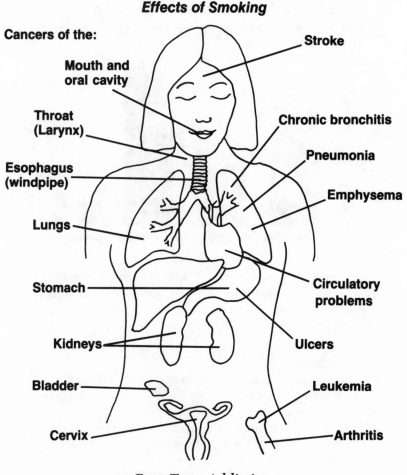

Part Two: Addiction

So now you are convinced you should stop smoking. You're in good company—so have the thirty-seven million people who actually have dropped the habit in the last twenty years. However, what keeps one in three Americans smoking today is a question of addiction, pure and simple.

You don't need lectures about an addiction you can't help. What you need are some useful tools to help you break that addictive pattern, and give the single biggest boost to your longevity, vitality, and health. That means understanding your physiological relation to smoking—what it does to your body's biochemistry.

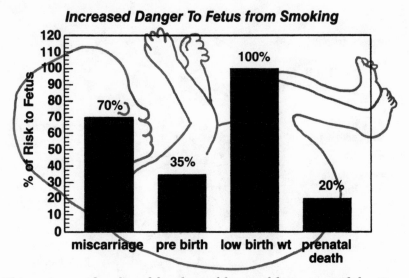

Increased Danger To Fetus from Smoking

This quiz was developed by the Public Health Service of the National Institutes of Health to help you gauge your nicotine tolerance.

NICOTINE TOLERANCE QUIZ

1. How soon after wakening do you first light a cigarette?
   A. Within 30 minutes
   B. After 30 minutes
2. Is it hard for you to obey the "no smoking" rules in areas like the doctor's office, theaters, or restaurants?
   A. No
   B. Yes
3. Which is the most satisfying cigarette you smoke all day?
   A. The first one of the day
   B. Some one other than the first
4. How many cigarettes do you smoke in a typical day?
   A. 1–15
   B. 16–25
   C. More than 25
5. Do you smoke more before noon than during the rest of the day?
   A. No
   B. Yes
6. Do you smoke when you are ill and staying in bed most of the day?
   A. Yes
   B. No

7. Is your cigarette brand's content of nicotine and tar:
   A. High (1.3 mg or more)
   B. Medium (1.0–1.2 mg)
   C. Low (0.9 mg or less)
8. Do you inhale?
   A. Never
   B. Sometimes
   C. Always

SCORING:

1 A = 1 point, B = 0 point
2 A = 0 point, B = 1 point
3 A = 1 point, B = 0 point
4 A = 0 point, B = 1 point, C = 2 points
5 A = 0 point, B = 1 point
6 A = 1 point, B = 0 point
7 A = 2 points B = 1 point, C = 0 point
8 A = 0 point B = 1 point, C = 2 points

Total: _____

If you score 6 points or more, consider yourself as tolerant to nicotine. For you, quitting may involve some degree of physical discomfort as your body adjusts.

If you score below 6 points, you are not likely to be physically addicted yet, so quitting should be easier.

Summary ▶ Knowing your physical tolerance is a necessary step so you know what to expect when you quit.

Part Three: What's in it for You?

Good—you have taken yet another step on your road to a smoke-free, youthful body. But as any smoker knows, physical needs are only a part of the picture. Now that you have assessed your physiological tolerance, this section will help you understand the psychological benefits you get out of smoking. The following is another test developed by the National Institutes of Health to help you do that. It is your next step. Make sure you answer every question by circling the number in the column that applies.

	Always	Usually	Sometimes	Seldom	Never
A. I smoke cigarettes to keep myself from slowing down.	5	4	3	2	1
B. Handling and touching a cigarette is part of enjoying smoking.	5	4	3	2	1
C. I feel pleasant and relaxed when I smoke.	5	4	3	2	1
D. I light up when I feel tense or mad about something.	5	4	3	2	1
E. When I run out of cigarettes, I can hardly stand it until I get more.	5	4	3	2	1
F. I smoke automatically, I am not always aware when I am smoking.	5	4	3	2	1
G. Smoking helps me feel stimulated, turned on, creative.	5	4	3	2	1
H. Part of my enjoyment comes in the steps I take to light up.	5	4	3	2	1
I. For me, cigarettes are simply pleasurable.	5	4	3	2	1
J. I light up when I feel upset or uncomfortable about something.	5	4	3	2	1
K. I am quite aware of it when I am not smoking a cigarette.	5	4	3	2	1

	Always	Usually	Sometimes	Seldom	Never
L. I may light up not realizing that I still have a cigarette burning in the ashtray.	5	4	3	2	1
M. I smoke because cigarettes give me a "lift."	5	4	3	2	1
N. Part of the pleasure of smoking is watching the smoke as I exhale.	5	4	3	2	1
O. I want a cigarette most when I am relaxed and comfortable.	5	4	3	2	1
P. I smoke when I am blue or want to take my mind off my worries.	5	4	3	2	1
Q. I get "hungry" for a cigarette when I have not smoked for a while.	5	4	3	2	1
R. I often find a cigarette in my mouth and don't remember putting it there.	5	4	3	2	1

For each category below, a score of 11 or more is high, 8 to 10 is medium, and 7 or less is low.

STIMULATION CATEGORY: Total your answers to A, G, and M. If the total is more than 9, you rely on cigarettes to stimulate and enliven you, to help you work, organize, or be creative. You are a good candidate for a substitute of another kind of "high": five minutes of exercise in your office, a brisk walk.

TACTILE CATEGORY: Total your answers to B, H, and N. If the total is 9 or above, an important aspect of your smoking is the feel of it. Try substituting a pen or pencil, doodling, or occupying yourself with a small toy. You may want to squeeze a tennis ball or handgrip exerciser, or even hold a plastic cigarette.

PLEASURE CATEGORY: Total your answers to C, I, and O. A high score suggests that you are one of the people for whom cigarettes provide some real pleasure. If this is you, you are a particularly good candidate to stop because you can substitute other pleasurable outlets—reasonable eating, or social, sports, or physical activities—for smoking.

TENSION CATEGORY: Total your answers to D, J, and P. Those who score high here use tobacco as a crutch, to reduce negative feelings, relieve problems, much like a tranquilizer. You are likely to find it easy to quit when things are going well, but staying off is harder in bad times. For you, the key is to find other activities that also work to reduce negative feelings; dancing, meditation, yoga, sports or exercise, meals, or social activities work for many such smokers.

ADDICTION CATEGORY: Total your answers to E, K, and Q. Quitting is hard for those who score high in this group because you are probably psychologically addicted and crave cigarettes. You aren't likely to succeed by tapering off gradually. Instead, try smoking more than usual for a day or two, until the craving dulls, then drop it cold turkey, and *isolate yourself* from cigarettes for a long period. There is good news, though: Once your craving is broken, you are less likely to relapse because you won't want to go through that distress again.

HABIT CATEGORY: Total your answers to F, L, and R. High scores indicate that you are a "reflex" smoker. For you, quitting may be relatively easy. Your goal is to break the link between smoking and your own triggering events—food, a cup of coffee, sitting down to work. Think of tapering off gradually. Each time you reach for a cigarette, stop and ask yourself *out loud:* "Do I really want this cigarette?" If you answer no, then skip it.

The higher your score in each category, the more that factor plays a role in your smoking. If you score low in all the categories, you probably aren't a long-term smoker. Congratulations—you have the best chance of getting off and staying off.

Combined high scores across several categories suggest that you get several kinds of rewards from smoking. For you, stopping may mean you need to try several different tactics. Being a high scorer in both TENSION and ADDICTION is a particularly tough combination. You *can* quit—many such people have—but it may be more difficult for you than for others. If you score high in STIMULATION and ADDICTION, however, you may benefit from changing your patterns of smoking as you cut down. Smoke less often, or only smoke each cigarette partway, inhale less, use tapering filters or low-tar/nicotine brands.

Summary ▶ Knowing why you smoke will help you know how best to stop.

Part Four: How Best to Quit

Just as people smoke for different reasons, they also stop for different reasons and in different ways. Today, the field of smoking cessation has become a whole new topic of study among behavioral psychologists, psychiatrists, and practicing physicians. The range of possible interventions is both broad and effective, so that virtually every person who is motivated can find a way to stop.

For instance, you may not have fully appreciated the staggering range of techniques and approaches that have been tried. All are available to help you stop smoking:

Nicotine chewing gum*
Graduated smoke filters
Hypnosis (group or individual)*
Education/motivation lectures*
Aversive conditioning
Doctor's intervention
Physician and psychologist intervention*
Medication
Educational
Self-help books
Audio and videotapes
Acupuncture
Individual therapy
Rapid smoking
Relaxation therapy
Electric shock therapy
Satiation smoking*
Group counseling
Stress management

Biofeedback
No-smoking clinics
No-smoking contracts

Hundreds of test studies have shown that most of these methods help between one third and one half of their subjects to stop smoking. Only a handful of methods, those I have marked with an asterisk, seem to show greater-than-average effectiveness. Through all this research, several principles have become clear:

1. Different ways work for different people.
2. The best ways tend to combine several approaches.
3. Groups can be helpful.
4. If you can stay off cigarettes for a year, you probably won't relapse.
5. If you are sufficiently motivated to stop, you will.

Summary ► You can find an effective method to stop smoking.

Doing It Your Way . . .

Despite all these available avenues, research shows that most smokers simply prefer to kick the habit on their own, and that many millions have been successful doing so.

Here are the addresses of some of the best no-smoking programs and kits available, and those which you can usually obtain free of charge:

—The American Cancer Society—7 Day Quitter's Guide
3340 Peachtree N.E.
Atlanta, GA 30326

—Information Resources Branch
Office of Cancer Communications
National Cancer Institute
Building 31, Room 10A
Bethesda, MD 20892
or call: 1 800-4-CANCER

—Your local chapter of The American Lung Association
(listed in the White Pages)
or:

The American Lung Association
P.O. Box 596DN
New York, NY 10001

You now possess everything that I can give you in a book to help you stop smoking. You have the basic information, data about your nicotine tolerance, a psychological smoking profile, and information about what means are available to help you stop. The next move is up to you. Take the single biggest step you can to promote your health, extend your life, and make sure the years you add to that life will be more worth living.

Keep in mind all you stand to gain:

—Better wind, stamina, and endurance
—Increased capacity for exercise
—Better and more restful sleep
—Fewer colds and infections
—Reduced respiratory symptoms (coughing, mucus, asthma)
—Stronger heart and circulatory system
—Reduced unsightly aging of the skin
—Lower risk of cancer and debilitating disease
—More energy and vitality
—Extra years of life

I hope you will do yourself the biggest health- and youth-preserving favor you can. Make today the first day of your wonderfully long, wonderfully healthy, *smoke-free* life.

In review, the key points of this chapter are:

1. STOPPING SMOKING GUARANTEES BETTER HEALTH AND LONGEVITY.
2. KNOWING ALL THE FACTS IS THE FIRST STEP TO QUITTING.
3. KNOWING YOUR PHYSICAL TOLERANCE HELPS YOU KNOW WHAT TO EXPECT WHEN YOU QUIT.
4. KNOWING WHY YOU SMOKE WILL HELP YOU KNOW HOW BEST TO STOP.
5. YOU CAN FIND AN EFFECTIVE METHOD TO STOP SMOKING.

8

Keeping Your Bones Young

CAN YOU RECALL how it felt to move when you were young? Think back to a time when your every movement seemed free, fluid, easy. Your gait had a buoyant energy, your walk was steady and vigorous. You stood erect and alert, yet relaxed. It felt natural to bend, reach, and flex with easy grace. You took for granted an energetic strength. In all of your motions, from the smallest gesture to the most athletic jump, you felt a wonderful, free confidence, knowing that your body would do what you asked without complaint.

One of the joys of youth is that we enjoy every ounce of the natural physical grace that Nature designed into our bodies. Yet too often, we see that grace and flexibility diminish as we age. It may start with creaks and stiffness in the joints, or the twinges of an ailing back. Gradually you feel your joints become stiffer and less pliant. Maybe you cut down on sports or any activity that requires significant movement. No more can you count on bursts of speed, for you have lost confidence in how your body will react. With the passing of each year, you may watch the person in the mirror become more stooped; your walk becomes stiffer and more halting. As this continues, bit by inevitable bit, you will eventually take on the cramped movements, unsteady gait, and stooped posture of an old person.

It is a rare adult indeed in this country who does not suffer from one or more common skeletal problems, including the stiffness and swollen joints of arthritis, the debilitating agony of lower back pain, or the bone-wasting syndrome of osteoporosis.

But that doesn't have to be your future. And it won't be because this chapter includes the four key "bone-builder" steps you need to keep your bones healthy, hard, and young for decades to come. These steps will help you prevent or forestall common degenerative problems that weaken your body's bony frame. These bone builders are your key to maintaining strength and youthful fitness, increasing your ease of movement, and generally keeping your frame young and supple. More than that, they are your assurance that you will retain the lively walk, grace of movement, and general vigor that spells YOUTH.

Modern laboratory research on nutrients and cell chemistry suggests that most skeletal aging that occurs is not only preventable but reversible. Scientists are learning how to keep our musculoskeletal system strong and supple far longer than we ever thought possible. With the right care and attention, you can expect to stay spry and active into your sixth, seventh, and eighth decades of life. However, to enjoy that kind of health twenty years from now means you have to take simple steps today.

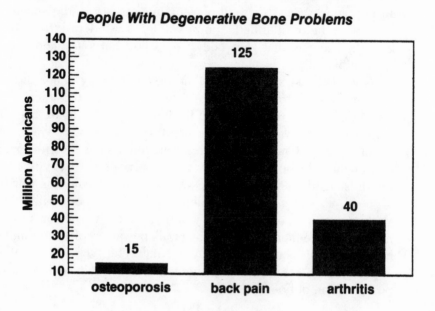

People With Degenerative Bone Problems

The Basics on Bones

You may think of your bones as the rock-hard, permanent supports for your muscles and organs. That is only partly true. Biologically your bones are more like bank accounts in a constant state of shifting deposits and withdrawals. But instead of money, they bank the minerals your body needs: calcium, magnesium, phosphorus, silicon, fluoride, and copper.

If you are in your midtwenties, those accounts are currently the strongest, and most mineral-rich, they will ever be. But by age forty, both men and women become less efficient at absorbing mineral nutrients from food. By age sixty-five, your body is only

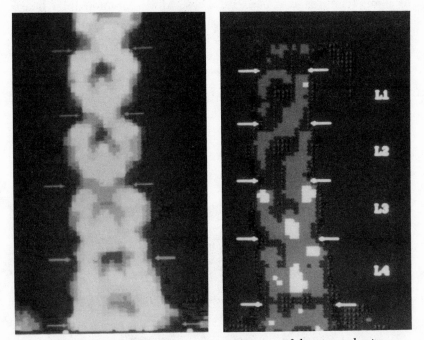

Bone scan of healthy spine.   *Bone scan of deteriorated spine.*
White areas indicate densest bone. Note how dense bone has virtually disappeared.

Dr. Chris Plato/NIA Gerontology Research Center

half as efficient as it once was. So, if it can't get minerals like calcium, magnesium, and potassium from the food you eat, it borrows them from your bones. As this borrowing syndrome continues, your bones become depleted, porous, and brittle, and you develop *osteoporosis*. Over a lifetime, this process can rob an average of 25 percent of your bones' density. *Bone aging is almost entirely due to the gradual loss of vital skeletal minerals.*

Porous bones age prematurely, collapsing and compacting. It becomes a particular problem in the spine; postmenopausal women lose up to 5 percent of spinal bone mass every year! Soon this aging actually shrinks the spinal column. By age seventy, the average American man can expect to lose as much as 2¾ inches in height; women, a less drastic 1⅞ inches. The change can be sudden: The collapse of one cervical vertebra can cost you an inch in height in a week! As the spinal vertebrae collapse, you start to show the dowager's hump, so often seen in older women.

Osteoporosis is far more than just a cosmetic problem. It leads to bone fractures that can cost lives. More common than heart attack, stroke, rheumatoid arthritis, breast cancer, or diabetes, this silent, bone-wasting disease is a leading cause of death in older Americans.

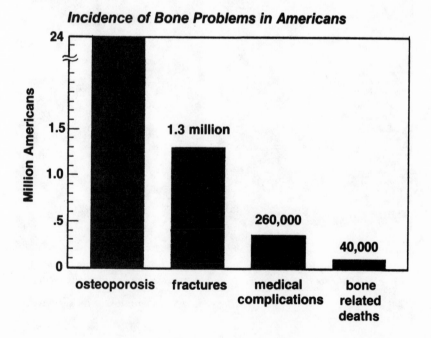

Incidence of Bone Problems in Americans

—24 million Americans have some form of osteoporosis (1 in 11).
—1.3 million osteoporosis fractures occur annually.
—1 in 5 of those fractures develop medical complications.
—40,000 of those fractures lead to death.

Remember: Since bone aging means loss of bone strength, rejuvenating your bones effectively makes your entire skeleton younger—and keeps you moving well, easily, and safely.

Are You at Risk?

In order to keep your skeletal frame as young and strong as possible, your first step is to find out if you are a likely candidate for premature bone aging and weakening. Do you fit into any of these risk groups:

1. Are you a woman?
2. Do you have small bones and a slight build?
3. Are you of Asian or Latin American heritage?
4. Do you smoke?
5. Did you have menopause before forty-five?
6. Do you have light (blond or reddish) coloring or hair?
7. Are your eyes any color other than brown?
8. Did you ever take oral steroids (such as prednisone) for more than six months?
9. Did your mother or sister break a wrist, hip, or vertebra other than in a serious accident?
10. Do you drink a lot of coffee or cola?
11. Do you get almost no exercise at all?
12. Do you get highly strenuous and prolonged exercise or have you ever exercised so much that you stopped menstruating?
13. Have you ever suffered from anorexia or dieted so much that you stopped menstruating?
14. Have you ever suffered from alcoholism?
15. Do you have a visible spinal curvature (dowager's hump)?
16. Do you now take, or have you routinely taken, diuretics, insulin, steroids, antiulcer, anticoagulant, or anticonvulsant medicines?

A yes answer to one of the above questions suggests you could be at risk for osteoporosis, but if you answered yes to two, three,

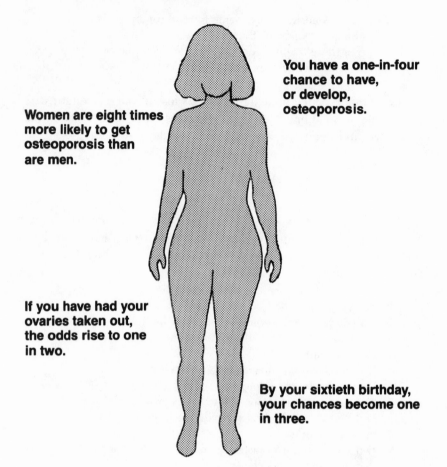

Women are eight times more likely to get osteoporosis than are men.

You have a one-in-four chance to have, or develop, osteoporosis.

If you have had your ovaries taken out, the odds rise to one in two.

By your sixtieth birthday, your chances become one in three.

or more of them, you should definitely begin incorporating the bone builder hints as soon as possible.

AS A WOMAN:

—Women are eight times more likely to get osteoporosis than are men.
—You have a one-in-four chance to have, or develop, osteoporosis.
—By your sixtieth birthday, your chances become one in three.
—If you have had your ovaries taken out, the odds rise to one in two.

Bone Builder Step One: Micronutrients

The first step to rejuvenating your bones is a micronutrient plan to make sure you get all the minerals and vitamins your body needs. The plan starts with two essential bone-building vitamins. They work in different ways to help your bones maintain their strong, youthful mineral balance.

Daily Bone-Building Micronutrient Mix

Vitamin C	1 gram
Vitamin D	400 I.U.
Vitamin B_{12}	100 mcg
Manganese	1 mg

Next comes *calcium.* I recommend:

If You Are . . .	*You Should Take:*
Male:	1,000 mg
Female:	
Teens	1,200 mg
Premenopausal/taking estrogen	1,000 mg
Postmenopausal or over 60	1,500 mg
In a risk group:	
Fair-skinned Caucasian	1,500 mg
Asian	
Small-boned	
Smoker	
Drinks much alcohol	
Pregnant or nursing, 19 and older	1,400 mg
Pregnant or nursing, younger than 19	2,000 mg

Remember: Just taking calcium alone is not enough to reverse bone aging. But it is an essential component of any bone-building plan.

Bone Builder Step Two: Eat the Right Minerals

The next step is to make certain that you get enough of certain bone-building minerals in the food you eat. That means eating a variety of whole foods that contain the following minerals to promote skeletal longevity.

Magnesium is a key bone builder. Unfortunately, most refined American diets are low in good sources of this vital mineral. Ironically, the diet your great-grandparents ate a century ago was two or three times richer in magnesium than diets today, thanks to all the magnesium-laden fresh vegetables and whole grains they ate. You should do the same.

Manganese also fights premature bone aging. I have listed some of the best manganese-rich foods below.

Boron. It is rare that we discover a wholly new nutrient, but that is what this bone-building mineral seems to be. The news on boron is by far the most exciting to appear on the bone-rejuvenation horizon recently. And recent it is—the pivotal findings about boron, its role in bone strengthening hitherto unsuspected, came just as I was assembling the research for this book!

A recent landmark study from the Grand Forks Human Nutrition Laboratory of the U.S. Department of Agriculture (USDA) shows that the mineral element boron, long overlooked, can play a key role in promoting and maintaining bone health—and in protecting our bones against aging and weakness.

This new bone builder is doubly powerful because it does double duty. First, it works as a team player, helping the body absorb other crucial bone-building nutrients from the food we eat. Research suggests that women who get enough boron in their food—3 milligrams per day, the amount you would get by eating moderate amounts of fresh fruits and vegetables—showed *significant improvement* in how their bodies absorbed calcium and magnesium. That means it works a bit like a catalyst—enough boron in your diet helps assure that your body will properly metabolize the other bone nutrients you need.

Boron also seems to work on another level, too. It can play a role in raising the levels of your hormones. This is helpful because these hormones, including estrogen and testosterone, are *directly related* to your bones' strength and resiliency. They are chemicals Nature uses to keep your bones healthy and young. That's why bone loss usually occurs after menopause, and why the most commonly accepted treatment for postmenopausal bone weakening is to prescribe female hormones. The hope is that boron may work to boost these hormone levels naturally, conferring the same kind of protection that hormone treatments would.

Because this news about boron is so recent, there is still much we have to learn about it. Laboratory scientists at USDA and elsewhere must determine optimal and safe boron-supplement levels. It may be that we can get enough boron from our diet, or that special supplements are recommended for people at risk for premature bone weakening. I expect that there will be a lot more news about this bone-longevity breakthrough appearing in research journals soon. I expect that boron will take its place in the bone-strengthening nutritional armamentarium within five years.

But you don't have to wait. You can start taking advantage of boron now—by including it in your diet, today. *The single best way to get enough boron* is to eat plenty of fresh fruits and fresh vegetables. They are Nature's prime, safe sources of this key bone builder. By eating a balanced diet of boron-rich foods, you can give yourself the same dose of boron that was used in the pioneering studies.

Below is a list of the best bone-building foods for an optimal balance of nutrients—including boron.

GOOD SOURCES OF:

Calcium: dairy products, low-fat yogurt, sardines (with bones), salmon, tofu, broccoli, spinach, collard greens, sesame seeds, seaweeds (used in Japanese cooking)

Magnesium: Dark green vegetables, broccoli, Brussels sprouts, spinach, dark-green lettuce

Manganese: Legumes, sunflower seeds, meat, dark-green lettuce, cloves, spinach, wheat germ, and black beans

Boron: Tofu, plums, peaches, grapes, raisins, apples, wine, prunes, almonds, pears, peanuts, dates, green leafy vegetables.

With all these minerals, the rule is "diet before drugs." Studies show that vegetarians suffer from osteoporosis much less than nonvegetarians. By including a good balance of fresh fruits and vegetables in your diet (which, of course, you are doing after having read the young-at-heart chapter) will automatically—and deliciously!—help your bones get enough of the vital minerals they need to stay youthful and strong.

Bone Builder Step Three: Nutritional Tips

In addition to eating the right foods, here are some special dietary tips to help prevent destructive bone aging.

—Eat a lot of fiber, but in natural, not supplemented, forms: whole grains, brown rice, oatmeal, and bulgur are better than refined wheat bran.

—Limit the amount of concentrated animal protein you eat. A very high-protein diet causes minerals to be flushed from the body—among them bone minerals. A more balanced, lower-protein diet helps guard against mineral depletion.

—Drink fewer carbonated drinks. They are acidic, which can upset your mineral balance.

—Both rhubarb and spinach contain oxalic acid, which can block mineral absorption.

—Reduce alcohol consumption to avoid flushing out minerals.

—Cigarettes have been shown to reduce estrogen levels and hasten menopause—another great reason to stop smoking.

—Avoid special very low-calorie diets, especially those with incomplete nutrients (weight-loss powders, drinks, or one-item diet programs).

Bone Builder Step Four: Exercise

Exercise is the vital fourth component to adding years to the life of your bones. It is now generally accepted that certain kinds of weight-bearing exercise are Nature's way of keeping your bones strong, healthy, and young. Check the guide on page 151.

If you are not now exercising, you should start gradually. Your goal should be to exercise for an hour or so, three to four times each week. Whether that means a session at the spa, a brisk after-

Weight-Bearing Exercise	Nonweight-Bearing Exercise
Impact aerobics	Biking
Basketball	No-impact aerobics
Dancing	Swimming
Football	Yoga
Gymnastics	
Hiking	
Lacrosse	
Running	
Skiing	
Squash	
Tennis	
Volleyball	
Walking	
Weight lifting	

dinner walk, or a racquetball game with a friend, you will be making an important contribution to your body's longevity.

But remember: Exercise by itself won't dramatically reduce the effective age of your bones. However, taken along with supplements and dietary bone builders, it is of vital importance to prolonging the life of your skeleton.

Your Doctor Can Help

The four bone-building steps outlined above will almost certainly help you rejuvenate your bones, lower the effective age of your skeletal frame, and protect against bone aging. But the key is to start the steps early enough in life so that your bones have not already started to weaken. However, since you may have already suffered significant bone aging, and so may need even more help, your doctor has a large array of treatments to reverse this age-related weakening. Treatment options include:

Time-release sodium fluoride
Fluoride calcium therapy
Estrogen replacement
Low-dose estrogen and calcium
Parathyroid hormone
Calcitonin
Growth hormone

If you follow the bone-building steps I've described, especially if you start now, the odds are you will never need any medical treatment because you will have effectively reduced the age of your entire skeletal system.

Good-bye, Creaky Joints!

Scientists have described some 110 forms of arthritis, all of which can contribute to premature aging, loss of mobility, and to a general feeling of being old before your time. Arthritis is the most common chronic disease in men, and the single leading cause of disability in old age. So, if you want to ensure yourself a more mobile, more active, more youthful life, there are some tips that can help keep arthritis at bay.

Keeping your joints young and pain-free requires two kinds of attention: physical and dietary. First, let's get physical.

It is the large, weight-bearing joints—knees, hips, and spine—that are most vulnerable to arthritis. That means you need to take special care during activities that use those joints, and this should be a focus of your arthritis-prevention efforts:

—*Sitting* places more stress and strain on the back than any other position. The basic law is: Don't sit longer than thirty minutes without getting up and stretching your back and legs. If your work involves sitting for long periods, make sure your chair supports your lower back, has armrests, and keeps your knees raised to a level slightly above your hips. If necessary, you may want to raise your feet on a small wooden box so that your knees are slightly higher than your hips.

—*Standing* can create joint stress as well. To relieve stress from standing, lift one leg so that hip and knee bend, and place one foot up on a short step or stool. After a few minutes, put that foot down and raise the other foot.

—*Lifting* often ignites serious lower-back pain. Always lift by bending your knees and keep your back as straight as possible. Try to lift and carry objects close to your body.

—*Sleeping* can be the most restful position for various joints if it is done correctly. Lie on your back with one to two pillows under your knees so that your hips and knees are bent, or on your side with hips bent so that your knees are pulled up toward your chest (fetal position), and with a pillow placed between your knees.

—*Muscles, ligaments, and tendons lose fibers with age,* which restricts the movement of your joints. One way to avoid damaging those joints is always to begin any strenuous exercise with a warm-up period of slow, easy, gradual stretches.

Diet also plays a key role in the joint pain that makes you old and creaky before your time. Your diet can help keep your joints young and supple in the following ways:

—Fish oils work as anti-inflammatory agents, helping alleviate the pain and premature aging of arthritis. Fish oils don't actually lubricate the joints themselves, but they chemically change the blood and reduce the body's own chemicals that lead to painful joint tenderness, swelling, and inflammation. Thus they break the chain of pain and inflammation that leads to arthritis. As we saw in the chapter on heart youth, you don't have to take fish oils in pill form; you will derive more overall benefit by eating fish. Certain varieties of fish have higher levels of the essential fatty acids that help protect your joints, Among the richest sources are: tuna, salmon, sardines, mackerel, sable, whitefish, bluefish, swordfish, rainbow trout, eels, herring, and squid.

—When it comes to keeping your joints young and agile, what you don't eat can be as important as what you do eat. It is clear that diet plays a role in preventing and relieving crippling arthritis pain. British researchers conducted a study on fifty-three patients with serious, crippling rheumatoid arthritis. When specific foods were eliminated from the diets of these patients, they reported "significant improvement" in joint symptoms. They had less morning stiffness, joint pain, and walked better. In other words—their joints and movement got effectively "younger."

I read about a mother of three children who suffered from progressive, crippling rheumatoid arthritis for some ten years. Then, her doctors asked her to abstain from eating dairy products, especially milk and cheese. Within three weeks her symptoms abated dramatically. For the first time in years, she was able to walk without pain, felt herself regaining strength in her hands, and could stop taking anti-inflammatory drugs. When, as a test, she started eating dairy products again, her severe arthritic symptoms returned within twelve hours. She has now been living symptom-free for several months.

You can put your diet to work in the same way to forestall the premature aging of joint pain. If arthritis is a problem, I suggest you avoid eating large quantities of foods in the nightshade family, since these are known to trigger or exacerbate joint inflammation. These foods include: zucchini, eggplants, tomatoes, bell peppers, white onions, potatoes, squash, and paprika.

—Incorporate this anti-arthritis formula into your daily plan:

Vitamin B_3 (niacinamide)	100 mg
Vitamin B_{12}	150 mcg
Vitamin B_5 (pantothenic acid)	250 mg
Vitamin B_6	100 mg
Vitamin C	3 grams
Zinc	75 mg
Evening primrose oil or linseed oil	Use in cooking and on salads

For a Better Back

You can't feel young with a crippled back. Today, 195 million Americans have had some back problems, and fully three in ten have a severe, chronic back ailment. These people know only too well that the agonizing pain of spinal or disk degeneration robs you of the freedom and movement of youth, casts a pall over your life, can even debilitate you.

To continue to enjoy the free and easy movement of youth during your whole lifetime, you have to avoid this most common crippling malady. What follows is a series of exercises and tips that you may want to incorporate into your daily regimen. These are used at the New York Hospital for Joint Diseases Orthopedic Institute, and were designed by Neil Kahanovitz, M.D., and Kathleen Viola, RPT. These exercises are your single best insurance against forfeiting youthful mobility to an aching back.

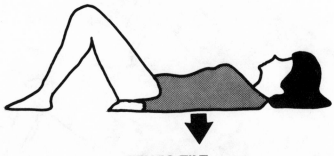

PELVIC TILT

Lie on your back, knees bent, feet on the floor. Tighten the muscles in your stomach and squeeze your buttocks together, pushing your back into the floor.

Objective: *to strengthen the lower abdominal muscles.*

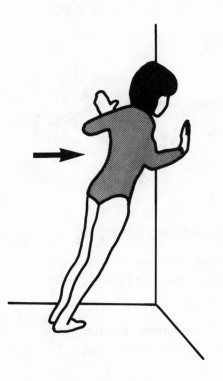

PECTORAL STRETCH

Stand facing a corner. Extend your arms and place your palms against the wall. With your body straight, lean toward the wall, keeping your legs straight and your heels firmly on the floor. Repeat, gradually increasing your distance from the wall.

Objective: *to stretch the chest and calf muscles.*

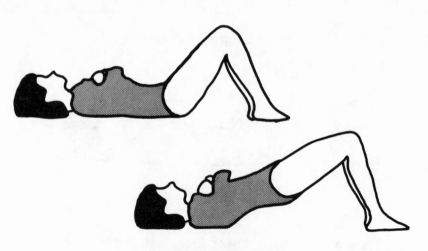

ARCH AND CURVE

Assume an all-four's position with your head in
neutral position. Allow your back to arch. Then,
curve your back upwards at the waist level, tighten-
ing your stomach muscles.

Objective: *to stretch and strengthen the back and
abdominal muscles.*

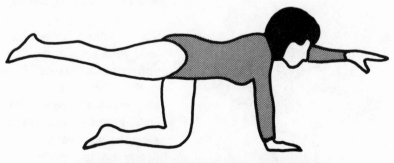

BACK STRENGTHENING EXERCISE

Assume all-four's position. Lift one arm and one
leg on the opposite sides, hold and relax. Alter-
nate sides.

Objective: *improve coordination balance and
strength of the back and supportive muscles.*

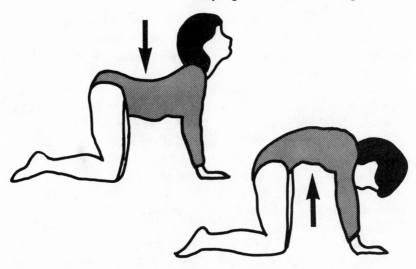

PELVIC LIFT

Lie on your back. Bend both knees so feet are flat on the floor. Squeeze your buttocks together and lift your hips off the floor.

Objective: *to strengthen the buttock muscles.*

At the Medical Frontier

Here are some of the most exciting research developments that will be available soon to help us protect and rejuvenate our bones and joints, so we can keep our body moving easily and well throughout life:

—*Screening tests for bone aging* are being perfected at Columbia University. A test, called a "GnRH-agonist test," has been developed that can reliably predict if a woman is likely to develop age-related bone wasting after menopause. The hope is that you could eventually get the test as part of a routine physical. A positive result would alert you and your doctor that special treatment is necessary to keep your bones young and strong.

—A tantalizing *bone-rejuvenation breakthrough* may depend on something as simple as the time of day, according to studies done by Dr. David Simmons, an orthopedic researcher at the University of Texas Medical Branch. There, doctors are exploiting the fluctuations of the body's own internal clock—what are called "circadian rhythms"—to keep bones at their strongest.

The researchers suspect that the peak time when the human body builds bone may be in the evening, before midnight. That's when the levels of crucial bone-forming hormones, such as para-thyroid and growth hormones, are at their highest. (As parents and pediatricians know, nighttime is also when children suffer most from the growing pains that are linked to bone growth.)

This suggests that drugs that help to increase bone growth, like testosterone and estrogen, or to inhibit bone shrinkage, like calcitonin, may work more powerfully during prime time than during the wee hours of the morning or during the workday.

These discoveries suggest that one common medication used to reverse bone aging builds more bone when it is administered in the morning, has little effect when taken at noon, and may actually decrease bone strength when taken late in the day.

The idea is so new that researchers are testing it only in lab animals, comparing a medication schedule of 8:00 A.M., high noon, and 4:00 P.M. If the animals show a difference in bone growth, the findings could be applied to humans, who could take a pill or even an inhalable spray of bone-strengthening drugs at the most propitious hours.

This simple discovery could prove to be one of those buried nuggets of medical lore that need only a perceptive medical mind to unearth them. If it proves out, it will be significant news on the anti-aging front. Simply watching the clock might give us a new, entirely cost-free way to avoid, and treat, bone aging. The sophisticated notion of cooperating, not competing, with the body's own internal hormonal rhythms may suggest that we should eat certain bone-strengthening foods at certain meals, to ensure that their nutrients are available when our body needs them most to build strong bones.

—A *new radiation drug*, dysprosium-165, promises relief to many of the six million sufferers of rheumatoid arthritis. Created by physicians in Boston, this short-lived, safe radioactive drug can be injected into damaged joints. It does with radiation what a surgeon would do with a scalpel, eliminating the damaged and inflamed tissue that creates crippling arthritis pain. Used in the knee joints, the procedure has relieved pain and restored free movement to more than three hundred patients so far, with virtually no side effects, for a fraction of the cost of surgery. It is now in clinical trials only in Boston and New York, but is hoped to become available to arthritis sufferers in fourteen major cities throughout the United States within the next year.

—In Israel an *electronic therapy,* called "transcutaneous electrical nerve stimulation," is being studied to relieve arthritis pain. It appears that the electrical fields diminish the body's inflammatory process in arthritic joints, and so reduce joint pain.

But remember: Rather than use such futuristic developments to remedy joint and skeletal pain, you can use the tips in this chapter to keep your bones and muscles young, supple, and strong—and avoid problems altogether!

9

Make Yourself Immune to Age

IF YOU WANT to assure that you live a long, healthy life, nothing is more crucial than your immune system. This network of blood cells, antibodies, and chemicals is your body's protection against the diseases that age us all. It fights germs, from common bacteria to exotic parasites to the deadliest viruses. It is also your sole guardian against the malignant, often deadly, growth of cancer. Your immune system is all that stands between you and diseases that can sap your energy, threaten your life, and make your body weak and infirm many years too soon.

Unaided, your immune system will lose almost 90 percent of its strength between the ages of twenty and seventy. As the years pass and those losses accumulate, your dulled immune defenses allow you to catch infections more easily. The body's energy is sapped in a chronic low-level fight against illness. As it weakens further, you may be one of the approximately seventy-five million Americans who will develop cancer in their lifetime.

Immune Rejuvenation means turning that process around. And you can. *There is no reason you can't have a superpotent immune system your whole life long.* By keeping your immune defenders intact and well armed, working at peak strength, you help make yourself "immune to age."

The steps in this chapter are drawn from several areas of research to help you do that. Some are based on the most complete findings about immune nutrients and anticancer diets published by the National Cancer Institute. Other suggestions in this chapter come from research being done, here and abroad, on how to strengthen the immune system of people suffering from the devastating disease AIDS. The "Antiviral Cocktail," which I will describe in this chapter, is based on findings from clinics and laboratories that show promise in helping strengthen the immune system. The intravenous vitamin C treatments are the ones that I am currently most excited about. Having used these with many, many patients, I have seen quite astounding results.

Together, these steps make up a solid prescription for immune longevity. That adds up to fewer infections, less debilitating illness, and less time wasted feeling sub-par. Immune Rejuvenation is your biological insurance policy that you will fight off disease, stay strong against cancer, and always enjoy the high energy and radiant health that Nature gave you.

That is 100 percent achievable if you follow the basic steps outlined below. Remember: You can give your body's disease-fighting troops a big advantage in their effort to keep you healthy and youthful, free of diseases and full of vitality.

The three steps to keeping your immune system young are:

1. Build *out* cancer from your life.
2. Build *up* your immune system to keep it young and healthy.
3. Build *in* added protection against disease-causing viruses.

Step One: Eat to Conquer Cancer

Believe it or not, you can conquer cancer in your life. Right now, statistics show that you have a three-in-ten chance of getting cancer during your lifetime, and that someone in your family has a three-in-four chance of being touched by cancer. With odds like that, you could well be among the almost one million Americans who will be diagnosed with some form of cancer this year. But if you could *remove* yourself from the list of "cancer candidates," this would give a tremendous boost to both your longevity and the quality of your life.

You can avoid being a "cancer candidate." The National Cancer Institute estimates that 80 percent of all cancers come from how we live. We know an *enormous* amount about how to build cancer risk out of our lives. According to the *New England Journal of Medicine,* diet is "second only to cigarette smoking as a determinant of cancer in this country." So, *just by eliminating cancer-risk habits, you can give yourself an 80 percent chance of avoiding cancer entirely.* This one step alone potentially offers you several extra decades of productive, healthy life. Yet despite all we know, only one American in seven has ever discussed with a doctor about putting these principles to work in his/her own life. In 1988 a survey showed that while 68 percent of Americans believe there is a link between diet and cancer, the great majority don't know what to do about it.

Fortunately, you don't have to count yourself among them. That's because many of the same health tips we have already discussed—your keys to rejuvenating your skin, heart, and bones—dramatically lower your cancer risk. If you are:

—Eating more fiber . . .
—Eating less fat . . .
—Eating more mineral- and vitamin-rich fresh vegetables . . .
—Stopping smoking . . .
—Moderating alcohol consumption to a reasonable level . . .

. . . then congratulations! You have already taken the most significant and positive steps to put cancer out of your life!

Of these health tips, reducing fat is particularly crucial. It has been shown that lowering cholesterol levels help the phagocytes, a vital type of immune cell, and that a generally low-fat diet not only reduces the free radicals that cause cancer, but actually helps the immune system work better.

You should know about one other important anticancer counsel. Make sure that you eat some of the following vegetables at least once each week:

Broccoli
Brussels sprouts
Cabbage
Cauliflower
Chinese cabbage

Collards
Kale
Kohlrabi
Mustard greens
Rutabaga
Turnips

New research shows that these vegetables, which belong to the cruciferous family, contain chemical compounds called indoles, which are thought to help reduce cancer, particularly colon cancer.

By making these changes in your living habits, you will be doing exactly what the nation's foremost cancer experts, from the National Cancer Institute to the National Research Council to the Surgeon General himself, recommend. Before long, you will begin to reap the benefits: a younger heart, cleaner arteries, and stronger bones. But the best benefit is to your long-term health and peace of mind, for you will have cut your vulnerability to deadly cancer by a factor of eight or more, and made a major improvement in the quality and length of your life! Amazing, isn't it, how changing a few health habits can do so much good to so much of your body?

Step Two: Your Personal Nutrition Plan for Immune Youth

A change of diet is half the cancer battle. The other half involves a pro-active, balanced supplement plan to make sure that your cellular defense system has all the micronutrients it needs to fight off cancer and keep part of your immune armies strong. One way to do that is with a balanced program of antioxidant nutrients, to fight the biological changes that damage your immune system. Clearly, a finely tuned immune system is essential to radiant health and long life. Which may be why women, who tend to have stronger immune systems than men, usually live longer.

Scientists at Memorial Sloan-Kettering Cancer Center in New York City have shown that nutritional deficiencies, especially of key immune-health nutrients, weaken the immune system. To keep your immune health at its youthful peak, your body's trillion or so immune cells need the right balance of vitamins, minerals, and amino acids. Yet study after study show that many millions of Americans are low on at least one key immune-boosting vitamin or mineral, like vitamin A, vitamin C, or zinc. It is no accident that the group with the lowest immune function—the elderly—is also the most likely to lack key immune nutrients. To avoid the premature aging that cripples so many people, here are the ingredients you need:

Vitamin A. Known to broadly strengthen the immune system, boost immune cells' reactions, and aid the body's fight against cancer, especially lung cancer. People who get more vitamin A have a lower incidence of cancer, and A specifically works as an antioxidant and anticarcinogen in the body. Instead of taking the pure form of A, which you can overdose on, I recommend beta-carotene, a harmless substance that your body converts into usable vitamin A.

Vitamin B$_{12}$ (cobalamine). One of the most important of the B-vitamin family when taken for immune health. It helps immune cells directly, and low levels are known to impair immunity.

Vitamin C (ascorbic acid). The number-one immune-boosting vitamin, C is known to increase several different kinds of immune-cell components, strengthen the cellular arm of the immune defenses, and increase production of the body's natural germ-fighting chemical interferon.

Vitamin E (alpha tocopherol). Plays a crucial role in preventing cancer directly, neutralizing cancer-causing chemicals, and generally boosting the immune system, according to research from Harvard Medical School, Tufts Medical School, the U.S. Department of Agriculture, and many other laboratories. It strengthens both arms of the immune system, protects against infection, and soaks up dangerous cancer-causing chemicals in your cells. High levels of E can reverse the age-related decline in immune strength, and low levels are associated with increased cancer risk.

Selenium. One of the two key mineral protectors against cancer, according to research being conducted at the University of California and the National Cancer Institute. Like vitamin E, selenium has been found to increase immune response, and people living in areas with sufficient selenium in their diets show a lower cancer incidence.

Zinc. The other primary immune mineral. The *American Journal of Clinical Nutrition* and researchers at M.I.T. have reported that zinc is necessary for the body's overall immune strength and that it seems to enhance the vital immune cells lymphocytes. In particular, zinc helps the anticancer activity of the body's immune T cells.

Organic germanium. A powerful immune stimulant long used by the Japanese, which has only recently been introduced into this country. It boosts the body's levels of interferon, increases several kinds of immune cells, including the body's natural killer and macrophage cells, and acts as an antiviral. It also has been found to fight tumors in both humans and animals.

Now, let's put that general information to work so you can *greatly extend your young and healthy years.* Each of the steps I have discussed includes a basic combination of key immune mi-

Youth-Preservation Immune Dose:	Your Correct Category:	
A	Beta-carotene	20,000 I.U.
	B_{12}	200 mcg
	Vitamin C	2,000 mg
	Vitamin E	400 I.U.
	Zinc	50 mg
	Selenium	100 mcg
	Organic germanium	150 mg
B	Beta-carotene	20,000 I.U.
	B_{12}	250 mcg
	Vitamin C	3,000 mg
	Vitamin E	400 I.U.
	Zinc	50 mg
	Selenium	150 mcg
	Organic germanium	200 mg
C*	Beta-carotene	25,000 I.U.
	B_{12}	300 mcg
	Vitamin C	4,000 mg
	Vitamin E	600 I.U.
	Zinc	75 mg
	Selenium	200 mcg
	Copper	0.1 mg
	Organic germanium	300 mg

Youth-Preservation Immune Dose:	Your Correct Category:	
D*	Beta-carotene	25,000 I.U.
	B_{12}	400 mcg
	Vitamin C	5,000 mg
	Vitamin E	600 I.U.
	Zinc	75 mg
	Selenium	200 mcg
	Copper	0.1 mg
	Organic germanium	300 mg
E*	Beta-carotene	30,000 I.U.
	B_{12}	500 mcg
	Vitamin C	6,000 mg
	Vitamin E	800 I.U.
	Zinc	100 mg
	Selenium	200 mcg
	Copper	0.2 mg
	Organic germanium	300 mg

*Important: For categories C, D, and E, take the dose for only three weeks, then go to category B for three weeks, then use category A levels for your maintenance dose.

cronutrients—vitamins, minerals, and amino acids. In Chapter 4 you established your Youth Preservation Category (see page 81). Use the level you achieved there to determine your correct immune-supplement regime.

"DRIP" Your Way to Immune Youth

Although most of this book is geared to things that you can do yourself at home, there is one powerful immune booster that you should know about, and that requires working with a physician. It is one I frequently use with my patients for its spectacular results in boosting immune function and effectively lowering immune age.

It involves many of the same immunonutrients listed in the table, but it is given in intravenous ("drip injection") form. The treatment has made a dramatic difference in a wide range of significant immune-related problems: the chronic, virally induced fatigue syndrome; the nearly ubiquitous infection of cytomegalovirus, which afflicts several million Americans; and long-term Epstein-Barr infection. These diseases can impair the absorption of vitamins, so that you are unable to take in the very nutrients you most need to fight off debilitating viruses.

To break this vicious viral cycle, a treatment was developed by Dr. Robert Cathcart, a pioneering orthopedic surgeon in California, who made his reputation as a premier orthopedic specialist at Stanford Medical Center. The treatment uses an injectable immune "cocktail" consisting of several key immune nutrients. I have found the best results by including vitamins C, B_5, and B_{12}, and zinc and manganese in the "cocktail." The elements must be carefully measured in appropriate proportions, and balanced and adjusted carefully to match the body's acid-alkaline chemistry. Then the mixture is gradually dripped into a vein in the arm. The treatment is painless, safe, and lasts only an hour or ninety minutes.

Similar intravenous immune-nutrient regimes are now being used internationally. Because these treatments can produce truly impressive changes in people's immune health, freeing them from chronic infections and illness, more and more doctors in the United States are using vitamin C intravenously in the fight against the immune-weakening diseases, including chronic viral infections, environmental and chemical allergies, AIDS, and cancer.

With my own patients, I have seen truly astounding improvements in overall vigor and health. They become seemingly younger and healthier in a matter of days with intravenous treatments. The results have brought about many complete cures among people who had tried numerous other approaches with no success. After a course of immune-boosting infusions, these patients have left my office, not only free of the viral disease that had plagued them for years, but with an immune system that is, in every functional way, stronger and dramatically rejuvenated.

I have taken drip injections to boost and strengthen my own immune system, and I urge you to think seriously about trying such treatments. If you are interested, look for a nutritionally aware physician in your area who can offer this nutrient-based intravenous approach.

Step Three: To Stay Young,
Vanquish Viruses!

You have already seen how to conquer cancer and boost your overall immune power. You have come to the final frontier of true Immune Rejuvenation: vanquishing the viruses that age you too soon and too fast.

Viruses play a large part in how and why we lose function and age too soon. Each time a virus makes us sick, it ages our body. In part, at least, the reason that we lose function with age has to do with an accumulation of years of viral insults. I can't count how often I have heard patients say, "I haven't quite been the same ever since I was sick last winter." You may have said it yourself, feeling that some part of your vitality has disappeared in the wake of an infection, mononucleosis, or even a bad season of the winter flu. You may have witnessed how a particularly serious illness can age a person shockingly fast.

We are learning, too, that viruses play a much larger role than we ever suspected in a wide range of diseases, including:

—Chronic-fatigue syndrome
—Leukemia
—Epstein-Barr syndrome
—Cervical cancer
—Uterine cancer
—Burkitt's lymphoma
—Liver cancer
—Lymphoma
—Meningitis
—Herpes
—Encephalitis

Each illness takes a little extra toll on our overall health, and makes us look, act, and feel older. That, in turn, leaves us more vulnerable to the next viral attack.

With viruses at the root of so many illnesses, it follows that *the best way to break that cycle is to protect ourselves against them, so that they don't make us sick and old before our time.*

"The Vicious Viral Cycle of Aging"

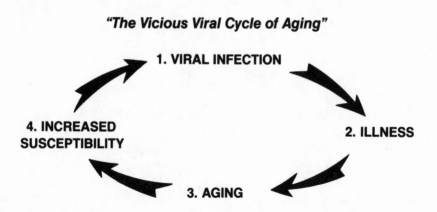

1. VIRAL INFECTION

2. ILLNESS

3. AGING

4. INCREASED SUSCEPTIBILITY

The best hope to do that comes from research on a new treatment for the deadly viral disease AIDS, and it involves a substance called "egg lecithin lipids" (you may also have heard it called AL-721). Developed in Israel, this food product—derived from three ingredients found in egg yolks—seems to work like a natural antiviral agent, helping to reverse the immune-system damage done by the AIDS virus. Some patients taking daily doses of the lecithin lipid paste report dramatic improvements in their immune system. It may work, in part, because it restores certain characteristics of young cell membranes and makes the cells' metabolism run more efficiently. There is much we still have to learn about the antiviral potential of lecithin lipids, and research is ongoing as I write this.

You don't have to have AIDS to put the antiviral power of this wonderful new treatment to work for you. Just as the "Antiviral Cocktail" shown below may work against the AIDS virus, it is believed to help control several other kinds of viruses—herpes, the ubiquitous cytomegalovirus, and the Epstein-Barr virus implicated in chronic-fatigue syndrome. Because all these viruses can damage your organs, sap your energy, and age you prematurely, it makes sense that an antiviral mixture can provide a good safeguard against their ravages.

Since the "Antiviral Cocktail" is made entirely from natural food products, it is very safe, and you can make your own "home brew" formula. For the lecithin, this version uses a soy product instead of cholesterol-laden eggs, and it doesn't carry a pharmaceutical brand name, but biologically it can be used as a generic, home-brew equivalent of the promising Israeli antiviral treatment.

Many of my patients have used this home-brew formula to derive many of the same beneficial antiviral effects of lecithin lipids. You should find that it can make a real difference in arming your body to fight the viruses that would otherwise accelerate your aging process.

"ANTIVIRAL COCKTAIL"

1. At a health-food store, purchase PC-55 lecithin, a high-strength soy-lecithin concentrate.
2. Add 1 tablespoon of PC-55 to 1 cup of orange or other fruit juice.
3. Let mixture sit 5 minutes, then blend until well mixed.
4. Add 1 generous tablespoon of olive oil or peanut oil, and blend thoroughly for several minutes.
5. The cocktail is best taken in the morning on an empty stomach. IT SHOULD NOT BE EATEN AS PART OF A BREAKFAST CONTAINING ANY FATS (eggs, whole milk, butter, margarine, cheese, or yogurt). You can drink it with fat-free cereals and 100 percent skim milk, or fresh fruit.
6. I recommend that you drink this mixture every third day. The vegetable oil should be kept in a refrigerator between uses. CAUTION: IF YOU HAVE CANCER AND ARE UNDERGOING TREATMENT FOR IT, OR HAVE HIGH CHOLESTEROL, YOU SHOULD NOT DRINK THIS COCKTAIL.

Tomorrow's Immune Health

By following the three-step process in this chapter—anticancer nutrition, immune boosters, and the "Antiviral Cocktail"—you will be doing everything now known about how to make your body's immune system younger, and your health more vital. Believe me, you will feel, and show, the results.

There is no other field where the changes are coming so quickly and dramatically as in immune health and rejuvenation. Among the developments that hold the most promise for the next five years:

—At Harvard University Medical School, scientists have created what they call "antibody bridges," molecules that work like tiny guided missiles, attaching one end of themselves to cancerous cells that the immune system may miss. These molecules then attach their other end to killer immune cells, forming a bridge between the immune cell and the cancer cell. Then the killer immune cells activate and destroy the cancer cells before they can grow into a deadly tumor.

—A major step in understanding the immune system occurred the week I sat down to write this chapter, when researchers at the University of California discovered a brand-new, unsuspected kind of immune helper cell. This fundamental biological discovery deepens our understanding about how the body fights bacteria and viruses, and will help us design more effective treatments against them and promote wound healing.

—One of the best immune boosters now under investigation may be entirely natural, cost-free, and wonderfully enjoyable: that old standby, the belly laugh. For years, there have been anecdotes and books suggesting that laughter helps boost the immune system. Two new experiments have helped lend scientific proof to that assertion. In one, researchers measured the levels of immune proteins in the saliva of people before they watched a film of a hilarious stand-up comedian. The researchers found that the immune factors, essential components in the body's first-line defense against viruses, rose dramatically after the subjects viewed funny videos, and stayed stable after they viewed more serious videos.

This finding coincides with other research showing that students who scored highly on questionnaires designed to measure humor have higher levels of virus-fighting antibodies in their saliva than do their more sober friends, and tend to react to a funny film with pronounced changes in antibody levels.

—One of the most intriguing avenues of research involves borrowing from Nature to restore youthful vigor and power to the immune system. The idea is simply to restore certain of the body's own chemicals, which are in abundance when the immune system is at its peak—in youth and adolescence—but which decline with age. Researchers at Veterans Administration hospitals in Wisconsin have found that the failing immune systems of elderly veterans are not fully capable of mounting a strong response when they are given seasonal influenza shots. However, their immunity was improved when the flu shots were "boosted" with a synthetic immune substance called "thymic hormone." This is based on a natural immune-boosting substance that a healthy body produces at high levels when young, but tapers off with age. Tests are under way to learn whether resupplying the body with this pro-immune hormone can effectively rejuvenate the age-weakened immune system.

Another hormone, called DHA, may also play a role as a potential immune regulator. At the University of Southwestern Texas Medical School, a researcher has already used it to extend the life spans of laboratory animals. This scientist took a breed of mouse with the inborn immune disease systemic lupus erythematosus, which usually begins to die after six months of life, and injected the mice with DHA hormone. About half the mice survived as long as ordinary, disease-free mice—*and even longer*. Other reports suggest that the same hormone also extends the life span of immunodeficient animals. The next step is to test DHA in animals with an AIDS-like immune condition. These studies offer hope that the answer to revitalizing the age-weakened immune system may be largely a matter of putting back hormones that age has taken away.

—Scientists have long argued that the blueprints for how we age are written in our DNA. They suggest that a genetic self-destruct mechanism built into our cells affects crucial bodily processes, creating aging and even death. If that is true, researchers hope, then we can isolate those genes and actually manipulate the aging centers that right now are ticking away in our body's cells. Researchers in Irvine, California, have taken a major step to doing just that. They have studied the genetic code of a simple creature, a roundworm, and have determined a single, crucial gene, labeled "Age-1 (hx 546)." When researchers changed that one gene and reimplanted it into a generation of worms, those worms lived two thirds longer than their ordinary siblings. That's the equivalent of a human being able to live 125 years! The research is a terrifically exciting first step, as it suggests where we can look to find similar genes in humans. One of the researchers predicts "a huge payoff twenty years down the road." The next step to be taken by the National Institute on Aging is to apply this same finding to other, more complex animals. If that experiment succeeds, it will bring us one step closer to being able to do it for the most complex animal of all—*you*.

10

Smart Beyond Your Years: Making Your Brain Younger

ANY ADULT WHO has spent time with teenagers can't help but feel a certain envy of their sheer, clear brainpower. At such a young age, before the predations of age, disease, and chemicals have set in, their minds seem to function at a biological peak. They work like natural learning machines, effortlessly absorbing facts and impressions instantly. Unlike adults, they rarely grope for a name or recollection. Their brains are razor-sharp and retentive; new intellectual challenges, whether learning a language or memorizing information for an exam, come with ease.

Few of us keep that keen mental edge. As the years pass, our mental faculties seem to lose their original power, clarity, and speed. Subtle errors creep in; a stealthy forgetfulness, a creeping inattention appear in our third decade. Names, facts, and ideas take longer to recall, and we cannot absorb, retain, and remember things in the same effortless way we once did. To ease the load on our mind and memory, we surround ourselves with various devices like Rolodexes, calendars, calculators.

But it doesn't have to be this way. By using the newest brain-youth tools you can do much to retain sharp, youthful brain and mental functions. A host of research teams has shown that you can bring your brain to its biological maximum, stimulate greater alertness, heightened concentration, and a surer, more confident

175

recall. With no pain and no expensive treatments, you can give yourself a functionally younger brain, regain the mental powers you once took for granted, and enjoy the benefits longer than you ever thought possible. That is, you can be smart beyond your years.

The real excitement comes when the experts show that it is possible to retain our intellectual faculties until a very advanced age, and even to reverse certain intellectual declines that have already started. Keeping your brain young is essential to reaping the rewards of an alert, enjoyable life. That is the life you deserve, brimming with interest, opportunity, and spice. The Youth Preservation tools that follow will help you keep your brain finely tuned, retentive, and sharp.

Young Between the Ears

You need to know something of the physical changes that occur in that gray globe between your ears as you age. Over the next few decades, your brain will shrink constantly. It will lose

 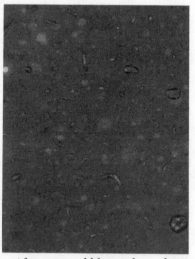

Brain section from a normal adult shows relatively uniform cells. *After aging, old brain shows degenerative deposits of protein.*

Albert Einstein College of Medicine

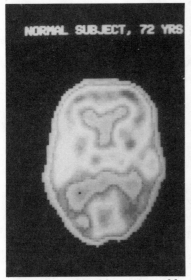

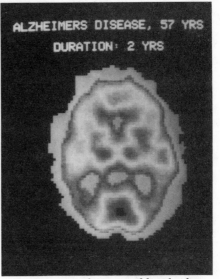

Brain scan of healthy 72-year-old. Bright areas show highest level of brain activity.

Brain scan of 57-year-old with Alzheimer's. Fewer areas of brain are active.

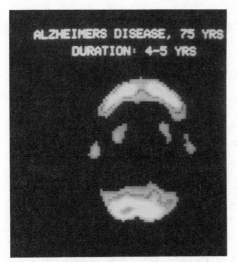

Severe Alzheimer's in 75-year-old. Note nearly complete absence of active brain areas.

National Institute on Aging

neurons, those connections between brain cells that allow you to think, feel, reason, even to understand the words on this page. By age seventy, most people have lost more than one billion of their ten billion nerve cells. By age ninety, some parts of your brain may have lost up to 40 percent of their nerve-cell connections!

Happily, though, we don't lose 40 percent of our brainpower. If we did, we'd be in real trouble. Nature has cleverly designed it so that as some brain cells die, the remaining ones actually expand, filling in and making new nerve connections to fill the gaps. The medical name for this process is "reactive synaptogenesis," or "resprouting," but you can think of it as just like a forest—as one tree falls, its neighbors expand, their branches taking over, enlarging to fill the vacant space. In the amazingly complex forest of your brain, that same process is occurring right now as new cells expand to make new connections and take over functions that are lost when old cells die.

New research has even indicated that the devastating changes of Alzheimer's disease may simply be an acceleration of the normal aging process that happens to us all—only the thinning out of the nerve synapses is magnified and speeded up to a tragic degree.

This means that the first step to keeping your brain strong and youthful must occur at a physical level. You must use diet and nutritional tools to slow the rate of the cellular changes in your brain, reduce brain-cell loss, and encourage regrowth of cells.

Step One: Food for Thought

It has been proven that nutritional status affects brain function. Therefore, the first step to keeping your brain working at full, youthful efficiency is to get adequate nutritional support. Here are certain nutritional basics to give your brain the maximum chance to stay young:

—High levels of dietary fat have been shown to lower brain function in animals—yet more evidence that it is a good idea to keep dietary-fat levels low.

—Antioxidants seem to play a clear role in keeping your brain at its peak. The brain has many fat-containing cells, which are particularly vulnerable to the oxidation damage caused by free radicals, which increase with age in the brain and cause certain brain-aging changes. A solid regime of antioxidants—beta-carotene, vitamins C and E, zinc, and selenium—can inactivate those destructive chemicals and prevent the premature aging of brain cells.

—Zinc is essential to the growth, development, and functioning of the brain. Levels of the mineral affect neurotransmitters, brain wave patterns, the brain's physical structures, even the thinking process. As brain cells are lost with age, they need to be rejuvenated, so adequate zinc is essential for lasting brain health.

—Lecithin is a food product containing choline, which has been shown repeatedly to improve mental-test results, help memory, and maximize brain function. In experiments, doses of choline made animals actually perform like much younger animals on mental tests! Lecithin seems to work by increasing one of the brain's key neurotransmitters, acetylcholine.

Of course, all these nutritional basics share one thing in common: You should already be following them. Zinc, lecithin, antioxidants, less fat in the diet—each of these counsels also appeared in the chapters on immune youth and cardiac rejuvenation. So, by following the programs already outlined, you will also be helping to keep your brain young—all with no extra work!

There are three other brain-boosting tips you should know about:

—The amino acid tryptophan helps the brain create serotonin, a necessary neurotransmitter involved in sleep, mental stability, coping with anxiety, and regulating pain. Many of my patients take a dose of 250 milligrams daily.

—The B vitamins—especially B_3, B_5, B_6, B_{12}, thiamine, and folacin—are critical to healthy brain functioning. They have been found to protect against mental slowness, memory defects, and mood disorders. Studies are now showing that deficiencies of B vitamins may impair recent memory, produce depression, create apprehension, hyperirritability, and emotional instability. These deficiencies appear to be much more common among older Americans than we have ever recognized. It may be more than a coincidence that this is exactly the group with the most serious problems in mental functioning. For that reason, I prescribe a solid B-complex vitamin supplement to many of my patients of all ages.

—Copper, iodine, and manganese are critical brain-nutrient minerals. They can affect brain functioning and mood, boost mental alertness and sharpness, improve memory, reduce nervous anxiety, and generally keep the mental status stable. Accordingly, make sure your diet includes foods that are a good source of these minerals, including dried beans, peas, shrimp, oysters and most seafood, seaweed, onions, whole grains (including the bran), green leafy vegetables, prunes, dark chocolate, seeds, nuts, fruits, and many other unprocessed foods.

Metals and Memory

Of course, not all minerals help the brain. The "heavy metals"—among them aluminum, mercury, lead, and cadmium—can be very toxic to the brain. Lead poisoning can cause mental sluggishness and even retardation. Cadmium can lead to significant memory loss and diminished mental function. Both aluminum and cadmium are thought to be factors in the tragic brain-wasting of Alzheimer's disease. Memory problems can be a symptom of heavy-metal poisoning, which you may be exposed to in many ways. Do you:

—Live in an area with a lot of environmental pollution, including smog or smoke?

—Live next to a major roadway or airport? German researchers have found that people living next to roadways have dangerously high levels of lead.

—Cook or eat food from aluminum pots or use aluminum foil? Certain acidic foods—tomato juice, lemonade, vinegar, orange juice—can draw the aluminum into them.

—Use ceramic bowls and dishes? Glazes used in some pottery can leach lead into certain foods.

—Have silver fillings in your mouth? Scientists in The Netherlands show that tooth fillings can release toxic metals into the body.

—Regularly take over-the-counter antacid remedies? If so, look on the label: One of the main ingredients is aluminum. If you've been taking them for a long time, you can be getting too much aluminum.

—Use an aluminum-containing antiperspirant? If so, you may be chronically absorbing excess aluminum through your skin.

If you fit into several of these categories, I recommend that you go on a special detoxifying regimen, in addition to the supplements we discussed earlier, to help keep your brain young and clear. This once-a-day, four-week program will help clear out heavy-metal residues before they can create a toxic buildup in your brain. Take

50 milligrams of glutathione
500 milligrams of cysteine

These amino acids bind heavy metals to help your body flush them out. The vitamin C and selenium that you are already taking will also help remove lead from your brain, and help your body eliminate heavy metals.

Step Two: Train Your Brain

The nutritional counsels above are only half the solution. With them, you have started to make your brain more physically youthful. Now comes the next step: to keep your brain young and to realize its maximum biological potential. That requires mental exercises and imagery to constantly train, expand, and hone the brain.

Modern research suggests that we need to exercise our brain to stay youthful and strong. We know that such training has a profound impact on how much, and how fast, our brain ages—or, better, on how young it stays. This process—termed "cognitive training"—is the best way to maximize our biological potential and keep our brain strong and sharp far longer than otherwise. The most exciting studies show that you can even *reverse* the brain's physical deterioration that may have already started!

—A score of research papers have shown that continual brain training and learning can offset and even reverse brain aging. Older animals that live in rich and varied environments, with the opportunity for constant learning, actually show organic changes in their brains. The nerve connections grow more complex, with more synapses, and more closely resemble the brains of healthy younger animals.
—A study of four thousand older volunteers showed that many of

them could greatly improve two kinds of brain skills that had declined with age, simply by using brain-training techniques. Two out of five subjects made so much progress that they actually regained the performance levels they had shown fourteen years earlier, in effect turning back the clock a decade and a half in their brain's functional age!

—A report by a National Institute on Aging task force showed that one in five older people with intellectual impairment may be able to reverse the downward slide.

—Cognitive training was found to increase older people's accuracy on standard mental-function tests, so they scored as though they were "younger."

The picture is clear: You don't have to lose brainpower as you age, and some of what you may have lost already can be retrieved and retrained. Rather, our intellectual skills, like muscles, seem to atrophy with disuse. Just as we need a physical workout, we need a mental one as well. With sufficient practice and stimulation, you can do much to reverse the "inevitable" mental declines of old age.

Putting It to Work for You

How can you take advantage of these new findings, and give your brain the mental workout it needs to stay younger, stronger, and more alert? One good way is by taking tests designed to sharpen specific skills of spatial orientation and inductive reasoning. Research suggests that practicing on such tests can help you sharpen those skills, and effectively lower the functional age of your brain.

Just doing these tests one time won't, of course, take years off the age of your brain. The key is consistency. You need to build into your life these kind of challenging mental exercises on a regular basis. There are several ways I tell my patients to do that:

—Get in the habit of doing games, tests, quizzes, puzzles, or brain twisters. You can pick up a collection at your local bookstore. Scrabble, word jumbles, acrostics, even crossword puzzles give the brain necessary exercise. Card games are particularly helpful for training reasoning and retention.

—Take a course at a local college or adult-education center. The practice you get in memorization, inductive or deductive reasoning, spatial orientation, or calculation will help give you the mental exercise you need.

—Pick up any one of the scores of preparation books for the SAT or other standardized scholastic tests. They are treasure troves of exactly the kind of varied, stimulating mental exercises that can help your brain stay young.

—If there is a university near you, its psychology department may have a specialist in psychometric testing. He or she may be able to help you obtain hundreds of brain-expanding tests and test instruments.

—Look in the "psychometrics" section of your local library for test instruments you can use as brain-training tools.

Step Three: "Memory Magnifiers"

There is no more important way to keep your brain young and powerful than to boost the power of your memory. Loss of memory is the first sign we associate with failing faculties, and a good memory is one of the most impressive aspects of clear mental functioning as we grow older. Happily, it is also one of the mental processes on which you can have the most significant, and dramatic, impact.

To boost memory requires no specialized tests at all. Here are four "memory magnifier" techniques that you can do on your own, as you go about your everyday life, with no tools or expense. Practice them and apply them diligently, and you can expect to see a dramatic rise in your retention and recollection abilities.

—*Mnemonics and acronyms* are the techniques of creating a word or sentence, each letter of which stands for one of the words you want to recall. Every Good Boy Does Fine has enabled countless music students to remember the letters of the treble clef musical staff E,G,B,D,F. This technique is used by every doctor to survive medical school. To retain the overwhelming crush of information physicians required—such as the names of the myriad nerves serving one part of the face—you make up a word whose letters are associated with each item. This technique works well with a shopping list, the names of your spouses or extended relatives, the signs of the zodiac, your boss's children.

—*Rhyme association*. Who can forget the first-grade spelling rule "I before E except after C"? And who hasn't reckoned the length of months by repeating "Thirty days hath September . . ."? The trick still works: Match an item you want to recall with a rhyming word, and you won't forget it. For best results, make up your own personal rhyme: ["Mish, mash, take out the trash."]

—*Visual association*. Pairing each item you want to recall with an associated visual cue is a powerful memory builder. You'll remember Mrs. Greenbottom, Mr. Brooks, and Ms. Burns much better if you turn their names into images. The more outrageous and improbable the images, the more firmly they will lodge in your memory banks. That's why I'll bet you remember Mrs. Greenbottom longest of the three! This technique also helps experienced card players recall the flow of cards. They create a visual image of which number cards in which suits have been played, then they recall, say, a gap in the lower middle of the spades, or a solid run in the face cards in hearts. With each new play, they adjust their internal picture accordingly. That way, they only have to remember four groups of one suit each, rather than fifty-two separate cards.

—*Loci association* is a well-proven memory-enhancing technique. To recall a list of things, you envision an area you know well. It may be your bedroom, your office, or your street. Then you mentally "place" each item on the list at a different spot in the familiar landscape. To recollect the items, you simply take a tour through that area, picking up each item as you see it. The technique works to organize any serial list: one's thoughts for a speech, Saturday's planned errands, or what you want to take on an upcoming trip.

The key in all of these techniques is the process of association itself. Memory is nothing more than associating the item we want to remember with a cue. Studies show that the more effort that we put into the act of perceiving or remembering something, the better we recall it. Your goal is to make that process conscious, pairing every item with a tangible and unexpected cue. Whether it is a rhyme, a word, a place, or an object doesn't matter. What counts is the effort you put into it. That's why devices you make up yourself work better than those you copy from others, and also why the best memory joggers are often the most outrageous ones.

At first, you may find this association process awkward, but it soon becomes second nature. As it does, you will notice a marked improvement in your memory. You will begin to make the physical changes in your brain's neuronal structure that strengthen memory. But most of all, you will give yourself a younger, more retentive mind, and reduce your effective mental age, making your brain younger in every sense of the word.

Looking Ahead—Super Brains?

Tomorrow's brain clinics may offer pills, shots, or treatments that greatly increase your brainpower, or at least help give the brain a chemical overhaul, restoring retention, alertness, and analytic capacity seemingly lost years before. Neurobiochemists are pursuing several promising avenues of research, including:

—The hormone DHEA may strengthen the brain as well, according to current research. Scientists surmise that DHEA is such a powerful bioregulator because the body can use it to synthesize more than a dozen distinct steroid hormones. In the brain, it seems to help cells grow in a more organized, interconnected fashion. Injected into test animals, it created dramatic improvements in their performance on laboratory mazes—in some cases allowing old mice, who had previously performed poorly, to run the mazes as well as young mice. It appears to work by helping the animals retain what they have learned from previous attempts.

—Test animals are getting smarter at the University of Rochester too, according to a paper published in the journal *Brain Research*. Neurochemists took rats with seriously failing memories and infused their brains with a chemical, norepinephrine, found in a normal, healthy brain. Immediately the rats began performing almost like much younger rats. To test the idea, the researchers then implanted into the rats' brains, cells that release the chemical. In several months, when the cellular transplants "took," there was a marked improvement in the rats' memories.

There is a feeling of great excitement in neurobiology laboratories around the country. There is a clear sense that we are closer than ever before to unlocking the chemical keys that will allow us to stay more alert, more retentive—just plain smarter—longer.

We may even be able to reverse the most common degradations in brainpower, keep a razor-sharp intellect and memory ten, twenty, or thirty years longer than we can today.

Until then, is there any way you can prepare yourself for these new findings? Absolutely. By giving your brain adequate nutritional support, in terms of micronutrients, vitamins, minerals, and amino acids, protecting it against accumulated toxins like heavy metals, and giving it the exercise it needs to stay young—in other words, by following the three brain-longevity steps in this chapter!

11

Can't Live Without It: Activity and Aging

Teach us to live that we may dread
Unnecessary time in bed
Get people up and we may save
Our patients from an early grave.
—British Medical Journal, 1947

A physically active life may allow us to approach our true bio-genetic potential for longevity.
—Journal of the American Medical Association, 1980

Suppose I told you that you have available *today* a powerful, proven method to stay young and vigorous longer. This single measure could ensure that for many more years you will meet life on your own terms, unencumbered by ill health or fading energy. It would help you greet each day with renewed energy and vitality, and give you the strength and vigor to do and be all you can. Even better, this technique is:

—Cost-free
—Enjoyable
—Free of special diets, treatments, or medication
—Easily incorporated into your life
—Guaranteed to have a positive impact on your health and longevity

The "secret" ingredient that makes this all possible? It is as simple as *regular physical activity.*

But you knew that, right? After all, we've already seen in other chapters how activity and exercise help the heart, circulatory system, and bones. But before you dismiss it as too simple, let's look at what you may *not* have known—because the news is just now breaking in scientific journals. Among the surprising and hopeful findings:

—There is a direct activity-longevity link.
—Your physical activity will determine your freedom from illness.
—There is new evidence on how much activity, and what kind, gives you the "longevity effect."
—You may need *less* exercise than you think to live better and longer.

Make no mistake: There is real news here. Most exciting of all, these findings represent a real advance from what we thought just a few years ago. I recall a recent newswire about a new medical advisory publication from the Canadian government. "If people are to live as long as possible without serious health problems," it said, doctors should prescribe exercise for patients. "The use of activity rather than bed rest in medical treatment is a real revolution in the 80's, . . . but doctors don't routinely prescribe exercise . . . because they just don't know." It may be years before this revolution trickles down to the average doctor's office, but there is every reason for you to put it to work *now* to feel, act, and look younger, longer.

All of this research boils down to a simple principle: Increasing your physical activity will add years to your life and life to your years, *even without strenuous exercise.* This short chapter reviews our state-of-the-art understanding of the activity-longevity link, and shows how you can use this knowledge in your own life.

The Activity-Longevity Link

For a long time, physicians have known that activity and exercise help specific parts of our body—the heart, the bones, etc. Now they have extended this research to show conclusively that *activity and exercise may be your single biggest defense against the changes of age.* To cite just a few voices from respected medical journals:

"Many of the changes commonly attributed to aging can be retarded by an active exercise program. . . . A high degree of physical fitness should offset age changes."—*Journal of the American Geriatric Association.*

"A portion of the changes commonly attributed to aging is in reality caused by disuse and . . . is subject to correction."—*Journal of the American Medical Association.*

"When people remain active, their body composition tends to resemble that of younger people."—*Handbook of the Biology of Aging.*

"Physical activity discourages disease, the absence of exercise invites disease."—*Predictive Medicine, A Study in Strategy.*

"Increased activity is associated with increased life expectancy. There is no doubt whatsoever that inactivity will shorten your life."—*The Physician and Sports Medicine.*

"Exercise results in improved survival . . . countering deleterious effects of a sedentary life."—*Society of Experimental Biology Journal.*

"By age 80 . . . additional life attributable to adequate exercise . . . was more than two years . . ." *New England Journal of Medicine.*

The latest research has proven beyond a trace of doubt what generations of mothers and gym teachers have long suspected: ACTIVITY IS LONGEVITY.

Not Just Longer . . . Better

Increased longevity is only half the battle. What counts as much as how long you live is how *well.* None of us wants to live for many years being feeble and doddering, our energy and faculties sapped. Our goal, rather, is to realize the longest possible "well-span"—years of being fully alert, energetic, and radiantly alive. I know your goal is to extend this period of life as long as possible, to keep the sparkle in your eyes, the spring in your step, and the joy in your heart for many decades to come. Plain and simple, it is your level of physical activity that will let you do that. If you want . . .

—Less chance of heart attack, chest pain, and artery disease
—Less likelihood of broken bones due to osteoporosis
—More muscle strength
—Less fat and more lean body mass
—More stable blood sugar
—More energy and better breathing
—Less joint pain
—More flexibility
—Less depression
—Better mental functioning, better memory, improved reasoning and confidence
—Better, more restful sleep

. . . then activity and exercise are the keys. A dramatic demonstration of how exercise makes you biologically younger was reported in the *Journal of American Geriatrics.* Doctors measured biological age through a common laboratory standard of the level of oxygen uptake of the lungs. They compared the scores of seventy-year-olds and younger subjects, who did and did not exercise, and found that when inactive seventy-year-olds started "moderate activity," their physiological profiles showed up to fifteen years younger. Those who continued to the "athlete" level of conditioning had a potential reduction of *forty years* in their age. It may be that the mythical Fountain of Youth is as close as the nearest health club!

If exercise rejuvenates the body, you'd expect inactivity to age it—which is just what studies show. When healthy people are forced to take bed rest or be confined, their biochemical profile starts to resemble that of someone much older. On certain physiological tests, people aged ten years during only thirty-six weeks of bed rest! Research with hospital patients, prisoners, and astronauts shows that inactivity takes a measurable toll on the immune system, the blood, cholesterol, heart function, bones, nerves, body composition, even brain waves. The moral is clear: Exercising is your best bet to stay supple, energetic, and alert, to keep your mood high, your muscles strong, and your mind clear. It is the best way to take years off your body's age, and to make sure that the years ahead will be the most enjoyable, vigorous, and healthy ever.

Be an Activist, Not an Athlete

By now, you know *why* you should be more active. For your life span, and your enjoyment of it, the benefits of increasing activity levels are beyond dispute. But wait just one minute, I hear you say. "Even if I have resolved that my days as a couch potato are numbered, I am also a far cry from being an athlete." Perhaps even the thought of running shoes makes you tired, and the idea of heavy, gasping, sweaty workouts makes you want to just curl up with a good book. You may be one of the millions who have tried exercising, only to give up in frustration after being unable to stick to a rigorous program. Does that mean you should turn to the next chapter and write off your chances for Youth Preservation through exercise?

Once upon a time, medical science might have said yes. But now I have good news—just for people like you. The latest research tells a very different, and much more hopeful, story. You may notice that throughout this chapter, I have referred to "exercise" together with "activity." Not long ago, the conventional wisdom held that one had to be a marathoner or a serious athlete, or at least a health-club habitué to gain longevity benefit from exercise. Exercise was thought to be an "all or nothing" proposition.

But the newest findings suggest that you can benefit, not just from grueling exercise, but also from more moderate levels of regular activity in your weekly routine. Just by increasing your basic levels of weekly activity, you increase your life expectancy. Conversely, says a Harvard Medical School researcher, "There's no doubt whatever that insufficient activity will shorten your life."

The key here—the real news you should know from the most recent findings—is that what counts is activity, not just athletics. Studies have shown that regardless of the strenuous exercise they do or do not get, men whose jobs require them to walk more, lift more, and generally be more active have fewer health problems and live longer.

These tidings mean that it's worth acquiring some new habits: Walk those extra few blocks to the store, take the stairs instead of the elevator, and do whatever you can to build-in occasions to be active rather than sedentary as you go about your daily life. Moderate activity will do. If you expend more than about 1,000 calories each week beyond your basic needs, you will cross the threshold to achieving better health and longevity. Best of all, think of all the pleasant ways to do that:

Gardening
Dancing
Playing with children
Riding a bike
Taking a Saturday hike
Going for a swim
Bowling
Chopping wood
Walking the dog

Even washing windows, scrubbing floors, and cutting the lawn—while not perhaps high on your "recreation" list—burn up calories and count toward your activity levels. Just think, this coming week you could make the house look terrific, treat yourself to an hour's walk afterward, play with the kids—and feel virtuous while doing it, knowing you are adding years—healthy ones —to your life!

This "activity revolution" provides real hope for a lot of us who may have sat out the "fitness revolution." *We who cannot dedicate ourselves to strenuous athletics can still reap many health and life-span benefits—just by staying moderately active.*

A few years ago, the Secretary of Health and Human Services issued a report showing that less than 20 percent of Americans exercise strenuously and often enough to meet popular aerobic fitness standards. Now we know that there is some hope for the 200 million-plus who haven't achieved star-athlete level of fitness training: For all the rest of us, then, these new findings offer great promise for longer, healthier lives.

Summary ▶ Regular activity, not just strenuous exercise, is the key to health and longevity.

Exercise and Mortality

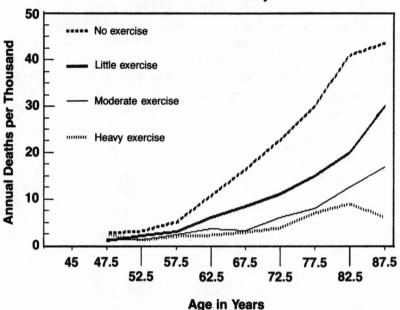

Feel Free to Exercise . . .

Although activity does more than we once supposed, I do not mean to discourage you from more intense exercise. It can extend your health and longevity benefits still further. This chart, based on epidemiological research, tells the whole story.

Certainly, those who get more exercise show the most dramatic improvements in longevity. But the real story is the one told by the rest of the curve. *The greatest benefits come when you change from no activity to moderate activity, rather than from moderate activity to high activity.*

Confucius said, "Every journey begins with a single step," and so it is with the activity-exercise continuum. If you are like most of my patients, you may find that by an easy increase in your general activity level, the next step gets easier and more pleasant. You may never end up a decathlon champion—but you will end up healthier and biologically younger.

That is really the moral of this chapter, and what I hope you take away with you. The more activity and exercise you get, the better (so long as you do not have physical limitations that make exercise unwise). But because you can't bench-press three hundred pounds doesn't mean you can't start increasing your levels of basic daily activity. Keep in mind that regular activity is just as important as hard exercise—and for many of us, much more realistic. So remember: Activity *is* longevity. To ensure yourself a long and healthy life, you really *can't* live without it.

12

Less Is More: The VLC Plan for Long Life

IF YOU ARE a seriously dedicated, die-hard Youth Preservationist, this chapter is for you. It is something of a "graduate course" in the ways you can preserve your youth and lengthen your life. The information it contains may not be something that everybody wants to use, but I do want you to know about it.

So far, we have emphasized those elements you need to *add* to your diet or life-style to live longer and feel much better. But if you were to ask virtually any reputable longevity biologist in any of the world's premier laboratories, you would soon learn that the greatest impact on your life may come, not from what you *add* to your diet, but from what you *subtract*.

All those eminent scientists know that there exists one undisputable, sure-fire route to preserving youth and vitality. It is one you can follow starting right now, and it is *virtually guaranteed* to add years, perhaps even decades, of healthy time to your life. Best of all, they would tell you, it is amazingly simple and costs you nothing.

You may be thinking that such a powerful technique must be a closely guarded secret, right? Not at all. It has been proven and reproven over more than fifty years of laboratory studies, published in hundreds of papers, proven and replicated around the world.

Does this sound too good to be true? It's not. Allow me to let you in on the "secret" the experts know. The single surest way to guaranteeing yourself a longer, healthier life span boils down to three letters: VLC, and they stand for Very Low Calories.

It is a scientific truism that *animals live significantly longer by dramatically reducing the number of calories they eat.* And the animal to whom that means the most is . . . *you.*

The experimental evidence for the VLC phenomenon is rock solid and beyond dispute. Among its astounding, proven benefits, such a diet:

—Extends life spans in lab experiments
—Lowers blood pressure
—Reduces destructive antibodies that attack the brain
—Reduces the loss of certain brain cells
—Strengthens the immune system
—Slows the aging process
—Lowers cholesterol and heart-disease risk
—Reduces muscle oxygen loss, and improves muscle function
—Reduces free-radical damage to the body's tissues
—Helps stabilize the blood sugar imbalance in diabetes
—Helps the body run at peak metabolic efficiency

Most dramatic of all, scores of studies show that animals on VLC diets live dramatically longer, without disease, with longevity increases of 50 percent, 65 percent, even 83 percent! In the words of one expert in the life-prolonging science of VLC diets: "Food restriction is unique in . . . the extent to which life is extended."

We do not yet understand just why and how a VLC diet prolongs life so dramatically. In part, it may work because it reduces body fat, which in turn diminishes toxic free radicals, and lowers cancer and heart-disease risk. But the longevity payoff of a VLC program goes beyond just these differences. Whatever the precise mechanism involved in VLC turns out to be, many generations of ancient, healthy laboratory mice are (long) living proof that it works!

VLC is not just a matter of eating "lite" foods, a few low-cal snacks, and skipping the occasional lunch. Not by a long shot. VLC diets that have been tested have involved a reduction in daily calorie intake down to about 60 percent of normal. In a typical group of test animals, this meant getting fed only every other day. It also meant they ate in such a way that vital nutrients were concentrated, and every single bit of food energy was used where it did the most good. As their reward for eating less and eating more efficiently, these particular animals lived 83 percent longer than their normal-feeding companions. In human terms, this would translate into living to the ripe old age of 137!

Of Mice and Man

Now you, of course, are not a laboratory mouse. But you don't need to be. If there is one thing all the experts agree on, it is the view expressed in one major paper, which reviewed a number of scientific studies on VLC diets: "The basic aging processes of all mammals are similar . . . nutritional manipulations that slow the aging process in rats will do the same in humans."

In other words, there is every genetic and biological reason to think that what works for laboratory animals works for the human animal. There is enough learned consensus that it will work for humans that several prominent gerontological scientists are enthusiastic about proposing VLC diets for humans. One eminent physician, a member of the medical school faculty at the University of California, Los Angeles, has been on such a very low-calorie longevity regimen for years—he is still going strong today and fully expects to enjoy buoyant energy and health for many decades to come.

Although the odds are that such a program works for the human animal, for most of us the problem is one of motivation. Few of us are eager to cut our diet so deeply. (I can hardly imagine anyone eager to go on an every-other-day eating program!) In order to get the maximum longevity benefit, and match the dramatic results of those studies, you would eventually need to cut back to a level of about 60 percent of the calories you now take in. For women, who normally need 2,000 calories per day, that would mean gradually dropping to 1,300; for men, it would mean a reduction from 2,700 to 1,650 calories. Gulp!

But when it comes to a VLC program, there is a much *easier* way. I don't really recommend such a drastic calorie reduction, because I find it is simply too hard for people to stay on such a restricted diet. In addition, trying to keep track of actual calories can be a tedious and painstaking process. But since the calories you eat usually translate directly into weight, let your pounds be your guide. Find yourself on the VLC Target Weight Table on the opposite page.

Normally, you probably weigh approximately 20 percent more than the value shown on the chart. For example, a woman who is 5 feet 7 inches tall, between age 55 and age 64, might weigh 155 pounds—or 20 percent more than the values in the VLC Target Weight Table. In any safe and appropriate VLC program, your goal is to reduce your weight to 20 percent below what you usually think of as normal for your age and height—that is what the values in the chart represent. Obviously weight is not the only thing that counts—it is also important that you eat the right foods to give your body the longevity nutrients it needs.

Do You Have to Go "All the Way"?

Many of my patients want to know if there is some way to gain some of the longevity benefits without such a severe diet—and without being a mealtime maniac. They ask: "Is there any reasonable way I can benefit from the VLC effect that has helped those Methuselah mice?"

My answer is: "Absolutely." Even if you don't want to go "all the way" to a strict VLC diet, you can still use its sound biological principles to extend your life and improve your health.

The VLC diet is simply the logical conclusion of many of the ideas in this book. The basic anticancer, heart-smart, pro-longevity steps we have discussed so far—less fat, less meat, more fish and filling fibers, less refined sugar and alcohol, appropriate vitamin and mineral supplements, and regular activity—are all 100 percent compatible with reducing the body's excess calories. You may decide to shoot for a personal weight reduction goal of 5 percent, 10 percent, or 12 percent below your current weight—but whatever your goal, you cannot help but gain—in health and in longevity.

VLC Target Weight Table

YOUR HEIGHT		AGE				
		18–24	25–34	35–44	45–54	55–64
4' 10"	Women	92	99	107	106	108
4' 11"	Women	95	101	109	109	110
5' 0"	Women	97	104	111	111	114
5' 1"	Women	99	106	113	114	116
5' 2"	Men	104	111	117	118	117
	Women	102	109	115	117	118
5' 3"	Men	108	116	119	123	121
	Women	105	111	117	120	121
5' 4"	Men	111	121	124	126	124
	Women	107	114	119	122	123
5' 5"	Men	114	124	127	130	128
	Women	110	117	121	126	126
5' 6"	Men	118	127	131	134	132
	Women	113	119	123	128	129
5' 7"	Men	122	131	135	137	136
	Women	115	122	125	131	131
5' 8"	Men	126	134	139	141	139
	Women	118	124	127	134	134
5' 9"	Men	130	138	142	144	142
5' 10"	Men	133	142	146	148	146
5' 11"	Men	137	146	150	152	150
6' 0"	Men	140	149	154	155	154
6' 1"	Men	144	153	158	158	158
6' 2"	Men	148	157	162	163	161

Calculated from: U.S. Center for Health Statistics, North American Association Study of Obesity

The VLC High-Efficiency Diet

If you are interested in trying a VLC regime, there are three principles to remember:

1. In general, the fewer calories you eat, the more years you add to your life.
2. The less you eat, the more *efficient* your diet must be.
3. You must undertake such a plan gradually and correctly or you can do yourself more harm than good.

In other words, the best way to use VLC is with a little TLC—the Tender Loving Care you must have to give your body what it needs, while removing what it doesn't.

Six VLC Tips

If you are interested in trying a VLC diet, here are six primary principles to keep in mind:

1. *Make every calorie count!* EFFICIENCY is the name of the game in a VLC diet. With so many fewer allowable calories, those you do eat must give you the most possible nutritive "bang for your buck." Your goal is to assure that you get enough energy and protein to stay vigorous, and nothing extra. That means:

—NO refined or highly processed foods. Simple carbohydrates and sugars must be cut to an absolute low.
—Eat about 80 grams of protein daily, and make sure your protein and carbohydrate sources are as "pure" and fat-free as possible.
—Keep fat to a bare-bones minimum—*no more than 20 percent of total calories.*
—Eat no more than 300 grams of dietary cholesterol daily.

2. *Go for bulk.* It is easy to cut down on food if you eat things that help you feel full. You will want to balance your diet to include a lot of fiber and bulky foods—ideally those that pass through

your system undigested, yet give you a feeling of having eaten. As a goal, aim to eat at least 50 grams of fiber each day.

3. *Use a fullness enhancer.* Another way to give you the feeling of fullness you need to stay on a VLC plan is to use a substance like guar gum. Guar gum is nondigestible, nonnutritive, and comes in liquid form. Once in your stomach, it expands to help you feel full. I have put hundreds of patients on guar-gum supplements to lose weight—it is a crucial component in any VLC diet.

4. *Don't spare those nutritional supplements.* Because you are eating so little food, you could short-change yourself on essential vitamins, minerals, and amino acids. On any VLC plan, you must take a strong, wide-spectrum micronutrient supplement to make sure your body gets all it needs to stay healthy on a reduced calorie diet. Micronutrient supplements won't add to your calorie intake, but they will give your body the necessary nutritional support. You will find an example of such a supplement plan in Appendix B, to give you an idea of the optimal levels to use if you are on a VLC diet.

5. *Ease into a VLC program very gradually.* If you try to drop to 80 percent of your weight immediately, you will be ravenous for a few days, and then fall off the VLC wagon with a resounding thump. It is far better to reduce your weight in gradual steps. You may want to establish a goal of a pound of weight loss every two weeks for the first five pounds, then a pound a month until you get down to the proper VLC maintenance level. It may take some time to achieve your target, true—but it is the best way to ensure you will stay with the program. *A drastic and transient weight loss WILL NOT enhance your longevity or health, and it WILL make it harder to achieve your VLC target.*

6. *Prepare yourself for a change in your appearance.* Your VLC efficiency diet will cause a real change in your body. You will lose excess fat—in places you didn't even know you had it. As you become lean, your body's metabolism will adapt to your new dietary levels, becoming ever more efficient. Your body's engines will run more cleanly and efficiently, extracting maximum energy from every bit you eat. You should be prepared for the new, lean person that emerges.

For those of you who are sincerely interested in going on a VLC diet, I have included my own sample diet in Appendix C.

It brings you to a level of 1,600 calories for women and slightly higher for men, a significant reduction of calories—AND A SIGNIFICANT STEP ON YOUR WAY TO A LIFE-PROLONGING DIET!

One Final Note

Let's talk frankly. I understand that you may not want to undertake a difficult regimen like a full-fledged VLC diet. That's fine. After all, by reading this book, you have already taken steps to give yourself not just many more years of life, but *better* years of life. I can guarantee that you will enjoy increased benefits—in health, vigor, energy, and well-being—regardless of whether you go all the way and adopt a rigorous VLC program.

My goal in this chapter, like my goal in this entire book, is to tell you about what tools exist right now that allow you to make a real, significant difference in the quantity and quality of your life. In that spirit, I want at least to make sure that you know about the proven life-improving promise of VLC high-efficiency diets. But beyond that, the choice is up to you. Different tools work differently for different people, and I am not saying you have to put yourself on a severe VLC diet. You can take advantage of many of these benefits by going part way—that is, by setting your own personal VLC target. You may choose a weight goal different from the value in the VLC Target Weight Table, maybe halfway between the number on the table and your normal weight. What I do want you to understand is that *whatever weight reduction you make is a change for the better.* You will still derive real benefits from the program because every step toward your VLC target gives you greater longevity and health benefits.

That's what this book is all about: feeling better, looking better, living longer. These benefits can all be yours if you decide to make the "secret" of the high-efficiency, extra-longevity VLC diet a part of your life.

13
Reprogramming Your Aging Computer

YOU HAVE OFTEN heard it said that "you are only as old as you think you are." I prefer to phrase it slightly differently: We are as *young* as we think we are. When it comes to staying young and leading a full exuberant life, it is not just your brain that counts, but your mind. That may be the single most important element, and it is the focus of this short final chapter.

According to a new field of research that has opened up in the last few years, your mind may be both the simplest, and the most powerful, weapon in your fight against premature aging. This new discipline is called "psychoneuroimmunology," or PNI for short. It charts the links between what goes on in our mind—our emotions, attitudes, and beliefs—and the health and vitality of our organs and physiological systems. The goal of PNI scientists is to unravel the mind-body connection that has perplexed and tantalized humans for millennia. Over the next two decades, I believe, this discipline will hold the most exciting and promising keys to longevity and long-term health.

However, far more important is what it means for you right now. It offers you nothing less than the keys to reprogramming the master computer that is ultimately responsible for aging— your mind.

The last five years have brought a torrent of fascinating and exciting findings from PNI researchers worldwide. They have shown that:

—In both men and women, mental programming for hope, hopelessness, or depression affects one's chances of getting, and surviving, many kinds of cancer, including lung, breast, cervical, and skin cancers.

—The personality programming you received as a child can affect your likelihood of developing cancer later in life.

—Animals given control over their environment fight off tumors better and live longer than animals with no control.

—Institutionalized people who have more control over their lives show dramatic improvements in overall health, even reversing bodily changes due to aging.

—Personality type may play a role in a person's susceptibility to diseases like asthma, peptic ulcers, arthritis, diabetes, multiple sclerosis, even heart disease and cancer.

—Brain chemicals that regulate happiness, sex drive, mental functioning, sleep, depression, aggression, and all of our other brain functions, have been found to activate specific immune fighters such as scavenger cells, T killer cells, antibody-producing cells, and immune boosters like interferon and interleukin-2.

—Our immune system's strength reflects our emotional and mental coping mechanisms. Life-style and psychological stresses can weaken our immune defenses, increase the likelihood of catching infections, and raise our risk for many kinds of diseases.

—People with strong psychological coping skills have been found to have more powerful immune systems, and higher levels of killer immune cells, than people with poor coping skills.

—Grieving, stress, and depression have all been proven to lower your body's immunological fighter cells dramatically.

—Research at Vanderbilt University Medical Center shows that patients who are programmed to expect a slow recovery after surgery exhibit more physical problems, and those who expect to leave the hospital quickly are much more likely to.

—By programming themselves with mental-relaxation tools, people can lower blood pressure and reduce the frequency of heart-rhythm abnormalities.

—George Washington University physicians found that patients can use mental imagery to change the levels of certain immune cells necessary to fight cancer.

—It has been discovered that people with multiple personalities have dramatically different physical reactions with their different personas. The changes include tolerance to medications, eyesight and sensory acuity, allergies, right- or lefthandedness, and neurological characteristics. Mental programming for each personality transforms the same individual into many measurably different biological "beings."

The list of discoveries is long and varied, touching on virtually every aspect of our body's functioning. This information avalanche points to one inescapable conclusion. From our hearts and blood pressure to our immune system, from our resistance to the common cold or to the deadliest cancer, every bodily process responds to some conscious mental and emotional control.

Your mind is the computer that controls the biological processes that age you. Even more astounding, we have learned that each of us holds the tools to *reprogram that computer* so we can retard the aging process and extend our young, healthy years. This represents a mind-boggling scientific awakening. We are just learning to harness the mind's awesome potential. I have no doubt that this is the medicine that will be practiced in the twenty-first century—but you can start using it now.

Who's Running This Computer, Anyway?

Your body's master aging computer already lies within you, and it is running even as you read this. In fact, it is already executing a complex and detailed "program" that will control your rates of aging, of fitness, and health. Your longevity program is the sum total of your expectations about what the next half century holds for you. It includes how you envision what your state of health will be, what you anticipate doing and being able to do, how you expect to feel, what physical limitations you see lying ahead for you, even when you expect to die.

Unfortunately, if you are like most people, *right now, you are running a longevity program that is fatally flawed.* It's not your fault. One cannot grow up in our culture without "programming in" some very negative expectations about aging. We are surrounded by a national conspiracy to sell ourselves short when it comes to growing older. For example, you probably see yourself on a slow downward curve after the age of fifty. You expect to lose your faculties, feel less energetic, move more slowly and with less ease, get sick more often. Perhaps you've seen older relatives grow infirm and frail for the last decade of their lives, so you may anticipate that course for yourself. You probably plan to retire, have some leisure time, and then find yourself on a slippery slope where you sicken, weaken, and eventually die. I expect that you see each change in your bodily state as a part of a diminishing, inevitable pattern of decay. Such negative images surround us, reinforced by experiencing how people used to age in previous generations, and by the national media and a culture that disseminates much nonsense about what it is like to be on the far side of sixty.

The mind-body scientists have demonstrated that your mental aging computer commands many powerful ways to *make those expectations come true*—slowly, gradually, and inevitably—through its control over your bodily processes. And it will do it, unless you rewrite the program. Now, for the first time, you have a chance to take conscious control of this extraordinarily powerful anti-aging tool and put it on your side.

PNI has shown us that we have the ability to create a "longevity conspiracy," linking our mind and our body's physiological systems for better health, more vigorous years, longer youth. Science has given us the tools, and it is up to each of us to believe in them, stop selling our future short, and put them to work right now.

Four Steps to a New Longevity Program

Fortunately, there are some simple and easy ways to reprogram your aging computer. Because, sophisticated as it is, it only operates on what you tell it. If you repeatedly remind your computer that you plan to live a long and healthy life, and that frailty and decrepitude have no place in your life, it will react accordingly. Here is a set of positive visualization exercises to help you do that.

Longevity Visualization Exercises

I. RELAXATION IMAGERY

1. *Relax* two or three times each day, sitting calmly for ten minutes in a comfortable chair, with your feet flat on the ground. Imagine yourself at ninety, being active, energetic, full of life.

2. *Create* your own internal "movie" of how you want to feel. Picture yourself among friends, enjoying yourself, feeling strong and wise. Imagine being surrounded by many people who love you and value your long lifetime of experience.

3. *Repeat* twenty times in succession, twice daily, an affirmation like: "I feel myself getting stronger, healthier every day. I will live to be a healthy, vigorous ninety-eight-year-old."

II. LIFE GOALS

At least once each week, I hope you can take some time out to ponder the following topics:

—Give some serious thought to the most major life change you plan to make after age seventy. Will you continue to work? Will you volunteer to help people? Perhaps you will branch out completely and start something you have always wanted to do. Will your goal be to make money, to serve people, to have a very creative or helpful career? At what age do you expect to change? What do you have to do now to prepare for it?

—Draw a timeline of your life, numbering each decade. Put a short label on each decade, describing its main feature or accomplishment. Now place yourself along the line. Notice at what age you ended the line. Now extend it another twenty years, and fill in the extra decades with what you want them to hold.

—Sit down and write up exactly what you want to do to celebrate your ninety-fifth birthday. Where will you be? Who will you be with? What will be the most special thing about it? Figure out what kind of physical exercise you will enjoy most in the next twenty years, and in the twenty after that. Make a list of something special you want to do in each five-year period for the next thirty years.

—Contemplate which friends you expect to be closest to in your eighties. Sit down with them now and share with them your thoughts and hopes about what you will be doing together.

—Discuss with your family, spouse, or lover what you are looking forward to most about living another forty years. As ideas occur to you, describe in detail what you will be doing in the year 2025.

—Think about the young people now in your life. Imagine what wisdom you will want to share with them when you are ninety.

—Spend a moment thinking about the aspects of your life that will be better, more fulfilled, or more interesting thirty years from now.

—Think about where you expect to be living in your late eighties. Is there a part of the country or of the world where you have always wanted to live? At what age do you plan to move there?

—If you see a negative image about aging, say to yourself, "That doesn't apply to me, because I am going to be a healthy ninety-year-old."

—Contemplate the most exciting project you want to have accomplished by the time you are one hundred.

—Take a moment to sit quietly and relax, and decide what age—at least ninety—you expect to live until. Get used to that age and remember it every time you hear, read, talk, or think about the future.

These are just a few ideas to inspire your own creative efforts. Your goal is to replace every one of your current negative images about what the future holds with positive, health-affirming, longevity-boosting scenarios, in which you are active, energetic, and healthy. This may seem awkward or strange at first, but it will soon become automatic. What you want to do is reshape your expectations so that you continuously desire, believe, and expect the image of yourself to come true. Your mental computer will help make sure that it does.

III. Physiological Changes

These changes are designed to give you specific, concrete images to help specific physiological systems in your body.

1. Go back to the photographs we have seen in earlier chapters. They show changes of aging: in your skin, arteries, spine and bones, and brain.

2. In each pair of photographs, concentrate on the younger, health-ier image. For two minutes, visualize a positive change taking place in your own skin, arteries, spine and bones, and brain.
3. Visualize that image as many times as you can each day.
4. After a week, change to another image of another part of your body.

IV. Longevity Role Models

To remind you what your future could hold, I suggest you copy out this list and post it someplace where you will see it often:

Sophocles wrote *Oedipus at Colonus* at age 92.
Frank Lloyd Wright designed award-winning buildings into his nineties.
Armand Hammer, age 91, runs a multibillion-dollar empire and re-mains actively involved with United States-Soviet relations.
Bob Hope, age 86, entertains and travels around the world.
George Burns, age 93, appears in films and on television.
Claude Pepper, age 89, is now serving his *twenty-first* term as mem-ber of the U.S. Congress.
Martha Graham, age 95, continues her work as a choreographer.
Irving Berlin, at age 101, continues to compose music.
Louis Nizer, age 87, continues to win cases in his law practice in New York City.

These are the best reminders that we all can be candidates for this list in our nineties!

Remember: Your longevity program can only keep you as young as the expectations you feed into it.

14
Putting It All Together

A major objective now and in the future should be to maximize
health and well-being during our essentially fixed span of life.
—Dr. Denham Harman, gerontological researcher

WE HAVE COME a long way together since we began our journey
long ago on the deck of Ponce de León's ship. You now possess
Youth Preservation techniques and formulas to extend the benefits of youth in many of your body's vital biological systems. You
have improved your skin and appearance, your bones, muscles,
blood, heart, and brain. You have reviewed the benefits of exercise and activity, learned the principles of a VLC diet plan, and
gotten the tools to reprogram your mind's longevity computer.
That is a lot of learning, and a lot to be proud of!

We have covered a lot of ground, so it might be useful to
review the basic longevity steps, the key components in your
twenty-two–point plan to better health, longer life, and increased
well-being.

FOR A YOUNG OUTER YOU:
1. ASK YOUR DOCTOR ABOUT RETIN-A CREAM.
2. TAKE THE YOUTH PRESERVATION NUTRIENTS BETA-
   CAROTENE, VITAMIN C, and VITAMIN E.
3. KEEP OUT OF THE SUN AS MUCH AS POSSIBLE.
4. USE A WIDE-SPECTRUM, PABA-OXYBENZONE SUN-
   SCREEN.

TO STAY "YOUNG AT HEART" (CARDIAC LONGEVITY)
5. STOP SMOKING NOW TO REJUVENATE YOUR HEART
   AND LUNGS.

6. CUT SATURATED FATS TO A BARE MINIMUM IN YOUR DIET.
7. EAT FISH AS A MAIN MEAL AT LEAST TWICE WEEKLY.
8. EAT FIBER TO REDUCE FATS AND CHOLESTEROL.
9. TAKE TIME EACH DAY TO RELAX AND REDUCE STRESS.
10. DO MODERATE EXERCISE OR A BASIC DAILY ACTIVITY, SEVERAL TIMES EACH WEEK.

FOR YOUNG BONES (SKELETAL LONGEVITY)
11. USE THE DAILY BONE-BUILDING MICRONUTRIENT FORMULA.
12. INCLUDE THE NEWEST BONE BUILDER BORON IN YOUR DIET.
13. REDUCE ALCOHOL CONSUMPTION TO AVOID FLUSHING OUT MINERALS.
14. DO EXERCISES TO STRENGTHEN JOINTS AND BACK.
15. USE THE ANTI-ARTHRITIS NUTRITIONAL SUPPLEMENT PLAN.

STAYING "IMMUNE TO AGE" (IMMUNE LONGEVITY)
16. OBSERVE THE ANTICANCER EATING GUIDELINES.
17. CONSIDER INTRAVENOUS VITAMIN C TREATMENTS.
18. USE THE "ANTIVIRAL COCKTAIL" TO REDUCE VIRAL ILLNESS.

YOUNG BETWEEN THE EARS (BRAIN LONGEVITY)
19. FOLLOW THE FOOD-FOR-THOUGHT EATING GUIDELINES, INCLUDING ANTIOXIDANTS.
20. KEEP MENTALLY ACTIVE AND USE MEMORY MAGNIFIERS TO TRAIN YOUR BRAIN FOR LONG-TERM HEALTH.
21. CONSIDER GOING ON THE LONGEVITY-PROMOTING VLC DIET.
22. USE MENTAL IMAGES TO REPROGRAM YOUR INTERNAL AGING COMPUTER.

These twenty-two steps represent the most comprehensive, hopeful prescription available today for longevity. If you incorporate them diligently into your life, I am 100 percent certain that in twenty weeks, you will feel better, look better, think more clearly, and enjoy more energy and vitality. Best of all, you will have put yourself on the road to a significant longevity boost. Twenty-two steps, twenty weeks, can give you twenty months (or years!) of extra, *healthy* life.

Putting It All Together

Throughout this book, we have explored very concrete, very specific steps necessary to add years to your life. However, I don't want to leave you with the notion that your key to long and healthy life is twenty-two distinct, disjointed fragments. We are now at the point where we can put it all together—because you are, after all, more than simply the sum of your biological parts.

Keeping yourself young, beautiful, and vital longer is not a matter of checking items off a list, but of creating one healthy, unified whole.

We have examined various branches of health—immune, cardiac, skin, neurological, skeletal, and mental. It is true that each of those branches must be healthy for the whole tree to flourish. But as any gardener knows, the roots are as important as the individual branches.

In your case, the root of true, healthy longevity lies deep within your cells. All of the changes we have talked about, in one way or another, go back to that fundamental cause of aging.

At the beginning of this book, we discussed several theories of aging. The most compelling, the free-radical theory, suggests very clearly that the losses of age are due to accumulated damage to trillions of your body's cells. That accumulated damage is the real cause of aging—and the real source of potential longevity.

If you look back at the twenty-two steps outlined above, as well as reviewing many of the other counsels given throughout this book, most of them share one thing in common: *They help fight the basic aging processes in your cells.* They give your body the antioxidant nutrients it needs, and minimize your exposure to damaging fats, toxins, and ultraviolet light. They create an environment where your cells work cleanly, without interference, as Nature designed them. Taken together, they focus longevity changes where they do the most good: at the root of aging, in the innermost machinery of your cells.

It is no biological coincidence that several basic steps in your twenty-two-point plan work synergistically in several different parts of the body. Eating fiber has benefits for your heart, your blood vessels, and your bones; antioxidants help your immunity, your skin, and bones; exercise helps your heart and bones and brain; and so forth. When you bear in mind that each of these steps is aimed at having an effect at the basic level of your cells, it makes sense that they will improve many different aspects of your well-being.

It should be clear by now that there is no thirty-words-or-less formula for resetting your cells' innermost biological clock. As we have seen again and again, such a formula can never be just one simple answer, nor one magic bullet. If you could ask virtually any responsible thinker in this exciting field about what each of us can do *right now* to stay young, you would hear that it involves a combination of different interventions, programs, and practices. That advice is at the core of the twenty-two steps you have been given. These steps let you do everything possible *now* to rejuvenate and reenergize the systems that keep you young and alive—from the deepest cells of your long bones to the most hidden folds of your brain, to the outermost surfaces of your skin. Taken together, these twenty-two steps could quite possibly add twenty years to your life—years of healthy, energetic living.

Prepare Yourself for Tomorrow's Breakthroughs

There is one last thing to think about. Throughout this book, I have tried to keep you informed about the terrifically exciting news that is waiting just on the medical horizon. In the course of writing this book, several new major findings have been announced. Others, I'm sure, will have been announced by the time you read this. Such is the breakneck pace of change in the field of rejuvenation.

Does that make this book obsolete? Just the reverse. The twenty-two steps in this book will keep you in tip-top shape to benefit from new research breakthroughs. It will do you little good to pick up the morning paper on, say, March 4, 2003, and find out there is a new magic youth pill if you are already wasted from cancer, bedridden with heart disease, stooped over with arthritis and osteoporosis, addled with Alzheimer's disease, or debilitated by any of a host of other chronic and crippling maladies! The twenty-two points we've discussed are changes you can make *today* so you can keep in the youngest shape possible for what science learns *tomorrow*.

On a More Personal Note

I hope you will congratulate yourself on the changes you have made in coming this far. Give yourself credit for being smart enough to see that you *can* fight your own war against the decay of aging, and assure yourself of youthful energy and health. You already know you can make a real difference in your well-being and longevity by simply putting the knowledge you already have to work. That is the realization we started with in the first chapter, and it seems a fitting place to close this part of our adventure.

In truth, an adventure like this is never ended. Our only solid guarantee is that the Youth Revolution will continue, that discoveries will broaden, and that more and more people will wake up and start to follow the kinds of changes we have discussed. Until they do, you are in the vanguard of those making changes now to ensure dramatically more, and dramatically *better*, years of vigorous life.

My very personal thanks for coming this far on this exciting journey. Through these pages, you have joined the growing club of far-sighted visionaries who are smart enough to start putting these state-of-the-art ideas to work now. Together, we will finish the quest that our ancestors started so long ago.

I have no doubt that we will see wonderful research developments in the next five, ten, or twenty years. Best of all, you will have the satisfaction of being in the best possible shape to take advantage of them because of the changes you have already made.

I wish you luck, and I know you will not be sorry, for you now have the potential to live a better, more vigorous and healthy life than ever before.

To help you realize that potential, I want to extend you the special invitation below. I am planning to host a wonderful free party—a reunion for readers of this book—on New Year's Day in the year 2045 (that's a Sunday). So, put the date in your calendar now, stay in touch . . . and I expect to see you there, ready to dance.

Until then, be well, and be youthful.

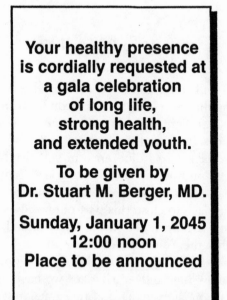

Appendix A

Sample Cardiac Longevity Menu

HERE IS A very specific five-day diet for a state-of-the-art heart. The low levels of fat in this menu are first steps to reducing the toll that age takes on your heart and blood vessels. If you wish to pursue this subject in greater detail, I refer you to my book *How to Be Your Own Nutritionist.*

Day 1:

Breakfast:

Low-sodium tomato juice
Whole-wheat toast with unsweetened jam
Low-fat yogurt with berries

Lunch:

Vegetarian chili topped with low-fat yogurt
Tossed green salad
Banana

Dinner:

Poached salmon
Brown rice and herbs
Salad of romaine lettuce, green peppers, tomato, alfalfa sprouts,
or: broccoli in garlic sauce
Pineapple spears and strawberries

Day 2:

Breakfast:

Bowl unsalted, unsweetened oatmeal
Skim milk
1 sliced banana or other fruit
2 slices whole-wheat toast or bran muffin
Herbal tea

Lunch:

Carrot and celery sticks
Sardines in tomato sauce
Whole-grain crackers
Peach
Skim or low-fat milk

Dinner:

Lean veal chops
Barley pilaf
Chicory and chopped celery salad
Steamed baby carrots
Broiled grapefruit

Day 3:

Breakfast:

Carrot juice
Whole-wheat cereal with skim milk
Blueberries

Lunch:

Low-fat cottage cheese with vegetables and kidney beans
Rice cakes
Nectarine

Dinner:

Vegetable sticks
Broiled brook trout
Parsleyed wild rice

Fresh spinach and garlic
Fresh fruit sorbet

Day 4:

Breakfast:

Low-fat cottage cheese
Grapefruit slices
Whole-wheat bagel

Lunch:

Hearty minestrone soup
Whole-grain roll
Skim or low-fat milk
Plums

Dinner:

Pasta primavera
Salad of tomato, cucumber, red onion
Poached pear

Day 5:

Breakfast:

Low-sodium tomato or vegetable juice
Oatmeal with cinnamon and apple
Skim or low-fat milk

Lunch:

Tuna-vegetable salad on whole-wheat toast
Lettuce and tomato
Pear

Dinner:

Broiled chicken
Baked potato with yogurt and chives
Salad of spinach, onions, carrots, mushrooms
String beans amandine
Kiwi fruit and berries
1 piece low-fat, low sodium cheese

For Dressings and Seasonings Use:

Vegetable oils
Low-fat yogurt
Low-fat cottage cheese
Vinegar
Lemon juice
Garlic
Onion
Herbs

Cardiac Longevity Foods

Foods That Preserve Your Heart	Foods That Age Your Heart
Fish high in essential oils:	
Salmon	Deep-fried fish
Mackerel	Fish in cream or butter sauces
Tuna	
Trout	
Haddock	
Cod	
Other fish:	
Sole	
Snapper	
Lean meats:	*Fatty meats:*
White-meat poultry without skin	Dark-meat poultry
Veal	Fried chicken
Lean beef	Duck
	Ham
	Pork
	Fatty beef
	Luncheon meats
	Hot dogs
	Bacon
	Spare ribs
	Lamb
	Sausage
	Liver
	Kidneys
Low-fat or skim dairy products:	*High-fat dairy products:*
Skim milk, or 1% or low-fat milk	Cream, regular milk
Farmer cheese	Half-and-half
Low-fat yogurt and cottage cheese	Nondairy creamers

Foods That Preserve Your Heart	Foods That Age Your Heart
Low-fat low-sodium cheeses	Regular yogurt
Park-skim ricotta	Regular cottage cheese
Part-skim mozzarella	Hard and semisoft cheeses
Ice milk	Ice cream, sour cream
Skim-milk buttermilk	Eggs

Fruits and vegetables:

Leafy green vegetables	Canned vegetables
Fresh vegetables	Canned fruits in syrup
Fresh fruits	Coconut

Grains:

Whole grains	Processed grains
Brown rice	White rice
Whole-wheat flour	Refined flour
Kasha	
Couscous	
Millet	
Bulgur	

Beans:

Pinto	Pork and beans
Navy	
Kidney	

Polyunsaturated oils:

Safflower oil	Saturated fats
Sunflower oil	Animal fats
Corn oil	Hydrogenated fats
	Coconut oil
Monosaturated oils:	Palm oil

Peanut oil	*Salts:*
Olive oil	
	Soy sauce
	Mayonnaise
	Pickled foods

Snack foods:

Chips
Candy
Cake
Pastry

Fiber Content of Common Foods

Food	Serving Size	Fiber Content (in grams)
Grains		
• Wheat bran	• ⅓ cup	• 6.5
• Oat bran	• ⅓ cup	• 4
• Popcorn	• 2 cups	• 3
Vegetables		
• Spinach	• ½ cup	• 6
• Sweet potato	• "	• 4
• Brussels sprouts	• "	• 4
• Corn	• "	• 4
• Baked potato (med.)	• "	• 3.5
• Turnips/rutabagas	• " (cooked)	• 3
Legumes		
• Lentils	• ½ cup uncooked	• 11
• Kidney beans	• ½ cup cooked	• 6
• Pinto beans	• "	• 5
• Split peas	• "	• 5
• White beans	• "	• 5
• Lima beans	• "	• 5
• Peas (green)	• ½ cup cooked	• 4
Fruits and Nuts		
• Apricots (dried)	• ½ cup	• 15
• Prunes (stewed)	• ½ cup	• 15
• Almonds	• ½ cup	• 10
• Peanuts	• ½ cup	• 6
• Blackberries	• ½ cup	• 4.5
• Raspberries	• ½ cup	• 4.5
• Prunes	• 4	• 4
Cereals		
• All-Bran (with extra fiber)	• 1 ounce	• 13
• Fiber One	• "	• 12
• 100% Bran	• "	• 9
• All-Bran	• "	• 9
• Bran Buds	• "	• 8
• Corn Bran	• "	• 6
• Bran Chex	• "	• 5
• Natural Bran Flakes	• "	• 5
• 40% Bran Flakes	• "	• 4
• Cracklin' Oat Bran	• "	• 4
• Fruit 'n' Fiber	• "	• 4
• Fruitful Bran	• "	• 4
• Shredded Wheat & Bran	• "	• 4
• Wheatena	• "	• 4

Appendix B

Sample Supplementation Plan for VLC Diet

ON A VLC DIET, it is essential to include a strong, balanced micronutrient-supplement plan. This ensures that your reduced level of calories will not lead to a deficiency of the vital micronutrient elements you need.

Vitamins:

Vitamin A	20,000 I.U.
Beta-carotene	20,000 I.U.
Vitamin B_1 (thiamine)	100 mg
Vitamin B_2 (riboflavin)	100 mg
Vitamin B_3 (niacin)	100 mg
Vitamin B_5 (pantothenic acid)	200 mg
Vitamin B_6 (pyridoxine)	50 mg
Vitamin B_{12}	200 mcg
Folic acid	400 mcg
Choline	200 mg
Inositol	200 mg
Biotin	100 mcg
Vitamin C	2,000 mg
Vitamin D	400 I.U.
Vitamin E	200 I.U.
Bioflavinoids:	
Rutin	400 mg
Hesperidin	400 mg

Minerals:

Calcium	400 mg
Magnesium	200 mg
Iron	10 mg
Zinc	50 mg
Selenium	100 mcg

Appendix C

Sample VLC Diet Plan

HERE IS YOUR sample menu plan for twenty-one days of a prolongevity VLC regimen. This plan is exactly balanced to give you the optimal mix of nutrients you need to take advantage of the strong life–span- and health-promoting benefits of VLC eating.

Be a bit generous with your servings of vegetables and salads, but be very stingy in using oil or fat in cooking or serving. If you do both those things, this plan provides approximately 60 percent carbohydrate, 20 percent protein, 20 percent fat—and for women, 1,600 calories each day. Men following the plan should eat the same foods, except they can increase their servings of salads and carbohydrates within reason, to allow for the extra calories the male body needs.

Day 1:

Breakfast:

2 large buckwheat pancakes, topped with berries and wheat bran
1 cup skim milk

Lunch:

Tuna salad made with:
water-packed tuna, celery, onion, low-fat yogurt on
2 slices whole-wheat bread
1 peach

Dinner:

Mixed salad with oil, vinegar, and herbs
1 large baked potato with low-fat yogurt and chives
3-oz chicken cutlet sautéed with peppers, tomatoes, and onion in very little oil

Snack:

4 rye crackers
Carrot sticks
Large apple

Day 2:

Breakfast:

½ grapefruit
1 poached egg
2 slices whole-wheat toast with unsweetened preserves

Lunch:

Vegetarian chef salad made with:
½ cup kidney beans,
½ cup chick-peas, oil, vinegar, and herbs
1 cup skim milk
½ grapefruit

Dinner:

Endive salad with oil, vinegar, and herbs
1 cup herbed brown rice
1 cup broccoli
5 oz poached salmon

Snack:

4 rice cakes
1 cup low-fat yogurt with strawberries

Day 3:

Breakfast:

1 cup cooked oatmeal
1 banana
1 cup skim milk

Lunch:

Tofu with bean sprouts, lettuce, and tomato on
2 slices whole-wheat bread
1 apple

Dinner:

Spinach salad with low-fat yogurt-based dressing with dill
Small butternut squash
1 cup French-cut green beans
4 oz lamb chop
1 whole-wheat roll with 1 tsp butter

Snack:

2 whole-wheat matzohs
A few almonds
1 orange

Day 4:

Breakfast:

Canteloupe wedge
Whole-wheat bagel with
1 oz melted low-fat cheese

Lunch:

Taco shell, stuffed with lettuce and tomato
½ cup beans
½ cup grapes

Dinner:

Mixed salad with oil, vinegar, and herbs
1 cup mashed potatoes
1 cup baby carrots
5 oz broiled sole

Snack:

4 Wasa crackers
½ cup low-fat cottage cheese
1 tangerine

Day 5:

Breakfast:

1 cup puffed rice with blueberries
1 cup skim milk

Lunch:

1½ cups minestrone soup
1 slice whole-wheat toast with
1 oz melted low-fat cheese
1 apple

Dinner:

Arugula salad with oil, vinegar, and herbs
1 large sweet potato with 1 tsp butter
1 cup Brussels sprouts
4 oz sliced baked turkey breast

Snack:

2 rice cakes with
2 tbs natural peanut butter
1 banana

Day 6:

Breakfast:

1 large bran muffin
½ cup low-fat cottage cheese
10 orange slices

Lunch:

Tomato stuffed with chicken salad
1 whole-wheat bagel
Mixed fruit with low-fat yogurt

Dinner:

Spinach salad with oil, vinegar, and herbs
1 acorn squash
1 cup cauliflower
5 oz broiled brook trout
1 whole-wheat roll

Snack:

2 cups air-popped corn
1 pear

Day 7:

Breakfast:

1 cup bran flakes
1 banana
1 cup skim milk

Lunch:

1 cup black-bean soup
1 oz low-fat cheese
2 slices 7-grain bread
1 tsp butter

Dinner:

Arugula salad with oil, vinegar, and herbs
1 cup rice
5 oz lean steak, with peppers, onions, tomatoes
1 whole-wheat roll

Snack:

Carrot sticks
A few cashews
1 small papaya

Day 8:

Breakfast:

1 cup cooked Wheatena
3–4 dried apricots
1 cup skim milk

Lunch:

Cucumber salad with low-fat yogurt and chives
2 pieces whole-wheat pita bread with
Hummus
Sprouts

Dinner:

Mixed green salad with oil, vinegar, and herbs
1 cup minestrone soup
Escarole
2 cups whole-wheat pasta and
Red clam sauce

Snack:

A few hazelnuts
1 banana

Day 9:

Breakfast:

Citrus salad
1 soft-boiled egg
2 slices whole-wheat toast with
1 tsp butter

Lunch:

1½ cups whole-wheat pasta salad with vegetables
1 cup cabbage slaw
2 rye crackers

Dinner:

Endive salad with oil, vinegar, and herbs
1 cup boiled new potatoes with 1 tsp butter and herbs
1 cup cooked spinach
4 oz grilled salmon

Snack:

4 rice cakes
2 oz low-fat cheese
3 dried figs

Day 10:

Breakfast:

1 cup puffed corn with blueberries
1 cup skim milk

Lunch:

½ grapefruit
½ cup low-fat cottage cheese with chopped vegetables
1 whole-wheat biscuit

Dinner:

Chinese vegetable soup
1½ cups rice
5 oz chicken cutlet, stir-fried with
Chinese vegetables

Snack:

2 whole-wheat matzohs
A few almonds
1 mango

Day 11:

Breakfast:

1 large oat-bran muffin with unsweetened preserves
1 cup skim milk
1 apple

Lunch:

1½ cups 3-bean salad on
Bed of lettuce
1 cup chilled steamed broccoli
2 rice cakes

Dinner:

Spinach salad with
Low-fat yogurt-based dressing with dry mustard
1 cup whole-wheat pasta marinara
1 cup green beans
5 oz veal cutlet with mushroom wine sauce

Snack:

1 cup low-fat yogurt with
Mixed fruit topped with
Wheat germ

Day 12:

Breakfast:

1 cup shredded wheat
1 banana
1 cup skim milk

Lunch:

2 slices 7-grain bread with
1 oz melted low-fat cheese
Lettuce and tomato

Dinner:

Arugula salad with oil, vinegar, and herbs
1 cup herbed barley and peapods
5 oz broiled mackerel

Snack:

4 Wasa crackers
Small amount of nut butter
1 apple

Day 13:

Breakfast:

1 cup cream of rye with
1 tsp butter
½ cup low-fat cottage cheese with herbs
1 orange

Lunch:

Tuna salad in whole-wheat
Pita with chopped vegetables

Dinner:

Mixed green salad with oil, vinegar, and herbs
1 cup lentil soup
1½ cups whole-wheat pasta primavera
2 pieces whole-wheat Italian bread

Snack:

½ cup low-fat cottage cheese with
Mixed citrus fruit
A few cashews

Day 14:

Breakfast:

2 whole-wheat waffles topped with
Low-fat yogurt and strawberries

Lunch:

Mixed green salad with oil, vinegar, and herbs
1 cup tabouli salad with a few pine nuts
1 apple

Dinner:

Endive salad with oil, vinegar, and herbs
1 cup zucchini and tomato
9 shrimp sautéed in olive oil and garlic over 1 cup rice

Snack:

4 rice cakes
1 oz low-fat cottage cheese
1 orange

Day 15:

Breakfast:

1 cup puffed wheat
1 peach
1 cup skim milk

Lunch:

Spinach salad with oil, vinegar, and herbs
1 cup rice with chopped vegetables
1 pear

Dinner:

Mixed salad with oil, vinegar, and herbs
1 large baked potato
1 cup wax beans
5 oz liver and onions

Snack:

1 cup low-fat yogurt with
Dried fruit and wheat bran
1 slice whole-wheat bread with small amount of nut butter
Unsweetened preserves

Day 16:

Breakfast:

1 melon wedge
1 egg yolk, 2 egg whites, as omelet or scrambled
2 whole-wheat biscuits with
1 tsp butter

Lunch:

1½ cups minestrone soup
2 pieces 7-grain bread with
1 oz melted low-fat cheese

Dinner:

Spinach salad with
Low-fat yogurt-based dressing with dry mustard
1 cup Italian green beans
2 cups whole-wheat pasta with mussels marinara

Snack:

2 Wasa crackers
Small amount of nut butter
1 banana

Day 17:

Breakfast:

1 cup Nutri-Grain
1 banana
1 cup skim milk

Lunch:

1½ cups vegetarian chili
1 oz low-fat cheese

Dinner:

Arugula salad with oil, vinegar, and herbs
1 cup buckwheat pilaf and corn
1 cup Brussels sprouts
5 oz red snapper

Snack:

2 cups air-popped corn
Celery sticks
A few cashews
3 dried figs

Day 18:

Breakfast:

1 cup cooked oat bran
1 apple
1 cup skim milk

Lunch:

1½ cups rice and beans with
Chopped vegetables

Dinner:

Mixed green salad with oil, vinegar, and herbs
1 large sweet potato
1 cup cauliflower
5 oz sliced baked turkey breast
Fresh cranberry sauce

Snack:

4 rice cakes
1 oz low-fat cheese
A few hazelnuts
1 pear

Day 19:

Breakfast:

1 large corn muffin
1 oz low-fat cheese
1 pear

Lunch:

4 oz sardines in water or tomato sauce
2 slices whole-wheat bread
Lettuce and tomato
1 orange

Dinner:

Endive salad with oil, vinegar, and herbs
1 cup broccoli
2 cups vegetable lasagna with low-fat ricotta
1 piece whole-wheat Italian bread

Snack:

½ cup unsweetened granola with
Dates and nuts

Day 20:

Breakfast:

1 cup puffed millet
1 nectarine
1 cup skim milk

Lunch:

Mixed salad with oil, vinegar, and herbs
1½ cups whole-wheat pasta salad with vegetables and
Grated low-fat cheese

Dinner:

Arugula salad with oil, vinegar, and herbs
1 cup rice and herbs
1 zucchini, steamed
5 oz broiled lobster tail

Snack:

4 rye crackers
Small amount of nut butter
1 apple

Day 21:

Breakfast:

1 cup cream of rice
3 prunes
1 cup skim milk

Lunch:

Large spinach salad with lemon and herbs
1 hard-boiled egg
2 slices whole-wheat bread
1 apple

Dinner:

Vegetable soup
1½ cups oven-baked french fries
3 oz lean hamburger
Whole-wheat roll
Lettuce and tomato

Snack:

3 rice cakes
1 cup low-fat yogurt
Mixed fruit

INDEX
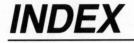

Z